Acknowledgements

This report was written by Bethan Emmett, with contributions from Duncan Green, Max Lawson, Belinda Calagues (WaterAid), Sheila Aikman, Mohga Kamal-Yanni, and Ines Smyth.

Special thanks to Belinda Calaguas, Nina Andrade-Henderson, Tom Noel, Kate Raworth, Arry Fraser, and Swati Narayan.

First published by Oxfam International in 2006 in association with WaterAid
© Oxfam International 2006

ISBN: 978 0 85598 569 1
ISBN Library Ebook: 9780855987756
Book DOI: http://dx.doi.org/10.3362/9780855987756

A catalogue record for this publication is available from the British Library.

Front cover image:
Proud Mum and Dad, after a routine maternity check-up at Machaze District Clinic, Manica Province, Mozambique.
Mother and baby are in good health.
Kate Raworth/Oxfam

Back cover image:
The world needs 4.25 million more healthworkers.
Helen Palmer/Oxfam

Reprinted in 2018
Reprinted by Practical Action Publishing Ltd
25 Albert Street, Rugby, CV21 2SD, Warwickshire, UK
www.practicalactionpublishing.org

Since 1974, Practical Action Publishing has published and disseminated books and information in support of international development work throughout the world. Practical Action Publishing is a trading name of Practical Action Publishing Ltd (Company Reg. No. 1159018), the wholly owned publishing company of Practical Action. Practical Action Publishing trades only in support of its parent charity objectives and any profits are covenanted back to Practical Action (Charity Reg. No. 247257, Group VAT Registration No. 880 9924 76).

Contents

Foreword

Acronyms and abbreviations

Summary
Public success: governments that ensure essential services for all 6
Public failure — when governments fail to act 7
Civil society: picking up some of the pieces 8
If the state is broken, the market does not solve the problem 8
What needs to happen 10
Recommendations 13

1. **Essential services: failing to meet essential needs 15**
Water and sanitation: far off-track 22
Health: enduring inequalities 22
Education: signs of progress 23

2. **What works? The case for universal public services 25**
Incomes matter, but policies matter too 27
When governments get it right: learning from success 30
Lessons from developing country success 32

3. **When it goes wrong: poor country government neglect and broken promises 39**
The missing millions — doctors, nurses, teachers, and administrators 44
Killer fees 46
Missing money 49
Servicing the rich 53

4. **Rich country governments: pushing for private provision and breaking aid promises 57**
Private provision is profitable, but not equitable 59
Things the rich countries don't try at home 65
Stealing staff from poor countries 67
Rich countries still falling short on aid 68

5. **Time to deliver: how developing countries and rich country governments can build effective public services 77**
What developing countries need to do 79
What rich countries need to do 94

Conclusion 99
Notes 100
References 113

List of tables

Table 1: Aid that is not co-ordinated does not get used 73

Table 2: Highly technical — rich countries that spend over 75 per cent of aid on technical assistance 74

List of figures

Figure 1: Missing the target: global progress towards the MDGs 20

Figure 2: Sri Lanka: less income than Kazakhstan, but healthier, better-educated people 28

Figure 3: Higher income levels do not always determine outcomes 29

Figure 4: Falling salaries 42

Figure 5: Missing teachers 44

Figure 6: Missing health workers 45

Figure 7: Minimum health spending: some regions are a long way off 50

Figure 8: Falling far short: missing money for the MDGs 51

Figure 9: Guns not schools — the ten worst offenders 52

Figure 10: Giving birth, rich and poor 54

Figure 11: Surviving childbirth depends on where you live 55

Figure 12: Broken promises on funding for essential services 69

Figure 13: Governments taking action, aid donors falling short 70

Figure 14: Some rich countries are progressing on budget support, most could do more 75

Figure 15: Abolishing fees gets education on the agenda and kids into school 85

List of boxes

Box 1: Public sector heroes 43

Box 2: Pay, or stay away 47

Box 3: Foot-dragging in some states is holding India back 55

Box 4: Uninsured and untreated in China 60

Box 5: The World Bank and the private sector 63

Box 6: NGOs working with governments — building services in Angola 66

Box 7: Take, take, take 67

Box 8: Dutch disease, or 'Is aid bad for you?' 72

Box 9: Community health insurance — a short-term alternative to user fees 86

Box 10: Getting involved — public participation in Porto Alegre, Brazil 89

Box 11: Government-led emergency human resources programme — Malawi 92

Box 12: How to support local government and build planning capacity 95

Foreword

By Mary Robinson
President, Realizing Rights: The Ethical Globalization Initiative
Honorary President, Oxfam International

A few generations ago, the poorer citizens of leading industrial nations had life expectancies not so different from those we see in sub-Saharan Africa today. It was only when public services for health, education, and water and sanitation were provided for all that life expectancies and what we now refer to as human development indicators rose sharply. Broad-based access to these social institutions has been key to the security and prosperity of people in wealthy nations, but we sometimes forget how recent a feature of society such public services are. Almost sixty years ago, the Universal Declaration of Human Rights affirmed that a decent standard of living, including access to health and education, were fundamental human rights. Subsequent international agreements legally committed governments to progressive realisation of social rights, including the right to water.

It is an important achievement that poor countries such as Botswana or Sri Lanka, in the space of only one generation, have been able to make progress in establishing basic public services that took over a century in Europe. How did this come about? The rights to education, health, and water have been promoted through free provision of public services. Everyone has gained, and in particular women and girls, with improvements in social indicators mirrored by greater respect for civil and political rights.

Public services for all people are well within our grasp: money and know-how are not what is lacking. Rather, political will is needed to challenge the status quo. We need to employ millions more health workers and teachers, and eliminate the fees that deny poor people the fulfilment of their rights. In developing nations, political leadership, government action, and robust public services are required. At the same time, the most important support that can be given by richer countries is long-term, predictable aid coupled with significant debt cancellation.

We know that clean environments, healthy families, and educated children are essential prerequisites to enable people to escape poverty. All governments must play their part to promote human rights, not only through effective judicial and political systems needed to ensure respect for fundamental civil and political rights, but also through guaranteeing strong and effective public services accessible to all, which are vital to the enjoyment of the rights to health, education, and water. As we move towards 2015, the target date for achievement of the Millennium Development Goals, we must take concerted action on this front.

Acronyms and abbreviations

ART	antiretroviral treatment
ARV	antiretroviral
BRAC	Bangladesh Rural Advancement Committee
DAC	Development Assistance Committee (of the OECD)
EFA	Education For All
FAWE	Forum of African Women in Education
FBO	faith-based organisation
FTI	Fast Track Initiative (Education for All)
GATS	General Agreement on Trade in Services (WTO)
GCE	Global Campaign for Education
GF	Global Fund to Fight AIDS, TB and Malaria
HIPC	Highly Indebted Poor Countries
IFC	International Finance Corporation (World Bank)
IMF	International Monetary Fund
MDGs	Millennium Development Goals
MIGA	Multilateral Investment Guarantee Agency (World Bank)
NGO	non-government organisation
NSP	non-state provider
ODA	overseas development assistance
OECD	Organisation for Economic Co-operation and Development
PEPFAR	(US) President's Emergency Plan for AIDS Relief
UNESCO	United Nations Educational, Scientific and Cultural Organization
UPE	universal primary education
VSO	Voluntary Services Overseas
WTO	World Trade Organisation

Summary

'*It was a miracle for us that free primary education came. Otherwise, John [aged 11] would still be at home.*'
Jane Nzomo, Kenya

'*Freedom translates into having a supply of clean water... being able to live in a decent home, and having a good job; to have accessible health care. I mean, what's the point of having made this transition if the quality of life of these people is not enhanced and improved? If not, the vote is useless!*'
Desmond Tutu, 1999

Classrooms with teachers; clinics with nurses; running taps and working toilets: for millions of people across developing countries these things are a distant dream. And yet it is these vital public services — health, education, water and sanitation — that are the key to transforming the lives of people living in poverty.

Building strong public services for all is hardly a new idea: it is the foundation upon which today's rich country societies are built. More recently, developing countries have followed suit, with impressive results. Sri Lanka, Malaysia, and Kerala state in India, for example, have within a generation made advances in health and education that took industrialised countries 200 years to achieve. Building strong public services is not a new idea, but it has been proven to work. It should be at the very heart of making poverty history.

In the twenty-first century it is a scandal that anyone lives without these most basic of human rights, yet millions of families still do. Today:

- 4,000 children will be killed by diarrhoea, a disease of dirty water
- 1,400 women will die needlessly in pregnancy or childbirth
- 100 million school-age children, most of them girls, will not go to school.

This report shows that developing countries will only achieve healthy and educated populations if their governments take responsibility for providing essential services. Civil society organisations and private companies can make important contributions, but they must be properly regulated and integrated into strong public systems, and not seen as substitutes for them. Only governments can reach the scale necessary to provide universal access to services

Meeting the MDG targets on health, education, and water and sanitation would require an extra $47 billion a year, compared with annual global military spending of $1 trillion, or $40 billion on pet food.

that are free or heavily subsidised for poor people and geared to the needs of all citizens — including women and girls, minorities, and the very poorest. But while some governments have made great strides, too many lack the cash, the capacity, or the commitment to act.

Rich country governments and international agencies such as the World Bank should be crucial partners in supporting public systems, but too often they block progress by failing to deliver debt relief and predictable aid that supports public systems. They also hinder development by pushing private sector solutions that do not benefit poor people.

The world can certainly afford to act. World leaders have agreed an international set of targets known as the Millennium Development Goals. Oxfam calculates that meeting the MDG targets on health, education, and water and sanitation would require an extra $47 billion a year. Compare this with annual global military spending of $1 trillion, or the $40 billion that the world spends every year on pet food.

Public success: governments that ensure essential services for all

To assess the performance of developing country governments, Oxfam has devised an Essential Services Index. This ranks countries in four social areas — child survival rates, schooling, access to safe water, and access to sanitation — and compares their performance with per capita national income. The comparison shows that some governments have consistently punched above their weights. Even though more than one-third of Sri Lanka's population still live below the poverty line, its maternal mortality rates are among the lowest in the world. When a Sri Lankan woman gives birth, there is a 96 per cent chance that she will be attended by a qualified midwife. If she or her family need medical treatment, it is available free of charge from a public clinic within walking distance of her home, which is staffed by a qualified nurse. Her children can go to primary school free, and education for girls is free up to university level.

Compare that with Kazakhstan. Even though Sri Lanka has 60 per cent less income per capita, a child in Kazakhstan is nearly five times more likely to die in its first five years and is far less likely to go to school, drink clean water, or have the use of a latrine.

Sri Lanka is not unique. Most recently, Uganda and Brazil have doubled the number of children in school, halved AIDS deaths, and extended safe water and sanitation to millions of people. In the Malaysian state of Pulau Penang, the public water utility company supplies water to over 99 per cent of the population and sets a subsidised price for the first 20,000 litres of water used by a household each month.

Successful governments have achieved results by providing universally available essential services which work for women and girls; abolishing fees in health and education and subsidising water and sanitation services; building long-term public capacity to deliver services; expanding services into rural areas; investing in teachers and nurses; and strengthening women's social status and autonomy as users and providers of services.

Public failure — when governments fail to act

'In the health centre they get annoyed when they treat you. If you don't have any money they won't take you. Then what? Well, you'll just be left to die.'
Marta Maria Molina Aguilar, mother of sick child, Nicaragua

For every Sri Lanka, there are other poor countries where millions of people cannot afford the fee to see a doctor, whose daughters have never been to school, and whose homes have neither taps nor toilets. In Yemen, a woman has only a one in three chance of being able to read and write. If she has a baby, she has only a one in five chance of being attended by a midwife. If she and her child survive childbirth, her child has a one in three chance of being malnourished and a one in nine chance of dying before their fifth birthday. If she lives in a rural area, her family is unlikely to be able to access medical care, clean water, or basic sanitation.

As well as devastating poverty, Yemen exemplifies the deep underlying inequality between the sexes: services routinely fail women and girls. Yet investing in women's welfare is the cornerstone of development – increasing both their life chances and those of their children. Across the developing world, women are more likely than men to fall ill, but less likely to receive medical care. They are expected to care for sick family members, but are often the last in the family to be sent to school and the first to be taken out when money is short. And it is — almost always, everywhere — girls and women who lose much of their day to hauling buckets of water over long distances.

The reality for the vast majority of poor people in developing countries is that public services are unavailable, or are skewed towards the needs of the rich, or are dauntingly expensive — and this drives up social inequality. Children still have to pay to go to school in 89 out of 103 developing countries, meaning that many poor children are forced to drop out of education. Most of them are girls. In one district of Nigeria, the number of women dying in childbirth doubled after fees were introduced for maternal health services. Deprived of public water services, poor consumers have to buy water from private traders, spending up to five times more per litre than richer consumers who have access to piped water. In many places, corruption is a major problem in both private and publicly provided services. Corruption and inefficiency mean patchy coverage, absentee staff, and charges for poor quality services.

In order to provide basic health care and education for all, the world needs 4.25 million more health workers and 1.9 million more trained teachers.

The public services that do exist are kept afloat by a skeleton staff of poorly paid, overworked, and undervalued teachers and health workers. Teachers' salaries in least developed countries have halved since 1970. And there are not nearly enough of these public sector heroes to go around. In order to provide basic health care and education for all, the world needs 4.25 million more health workers and 1.9 million more trained teachers.

Civil society: picking up some of the pieces

When their governments fail to provide services, most poor people get no education, health care, clean water, or sanitation. Those who do either have to bankrupt themselves to pay for private services or rely on civil society providers such as mosques, churches, charities, and community groups. These reach remote and marginalised communities and provide community-based services — for example, the home-based care for AIDS sufferers that has developed in hard-hit African countries such as Malawi. Informal provision of health care and education through local networks, often reliant on women's unpaid work, is common practice in many countries, especially for marginalised and vulnerable groups.

Civil society organisations can also develop and pioneer innovative approaches to service provision, and support citizens in claiming their rights to health, education, and water. But their coverage is partial, their services are hard to scale up, and the quality can vary greatly. In Zambia, for example, communities have clubbed together to build schools, but some of these lack even the most basic teaching materials and sanitation. The evidence shows that these kinds of citizens' initiatives work best when integrated into a publicly-led system, with their contribution formally recognised and supported by government. In Kerala state in India, and in Malaysia and Barbados, governments have built bridges to civil society, for example by funding the running costs of church schools, and have regularly monitored them to maintain standards.

If the state is broken, the market does not solve the problem

Market-led solutions have often undermined the provision of essential services and have had a negative impact on the poorest and most vulnerable communities.

Faced with failing government services, many have looked to the private sector for answers. Sometimes this has worked. Countries such as South Korea and Chile have achieved impressive welfare gains with high levels of private involvement in service delivery. But private providers are notoriously hard to regulate, and such services are prone to big inequalities and high costs and often exclude the poorest people, who cannot afford to pay for them. Market-led solutions have often undermined the provision of essential services and have had a negative impact on the poorest and most vulnerable communities. Water privatisation is the most notorious example, but under-regulated private sector involvement in health care in developing countries is also spreading rapidly.

- When China phased out free public health care in favour of profit-making hospitals and health insurance, household health costs rose forty-fold and progress on tackling infant mortality slowed. Services that were once free are now paid for through health insurance, which covers only one in five people in rural China.

- Chile was one of the first countries to implement private sector involvement in its health-care system. It also has the highest rate of births by Caesarean section in the world (40 per cent in 1997), largely because private hospitals have sought to maximise their profits from the extra costs of surgery and higher bed occupancy rates.

- Regulating private providers, especially powerful multinational companies, can be more difficult for weak states than directly providing services themselves. The global water market is dominated by a handful of US, French, and UK companies, such as Bechtel, Suez, and Biwater: the contracts they negotiate often 'cherry pick' the most profitable market segments, require guaranteed profit margins, and are denominated in dollars. If governments try to terminate these contracts, they risk being sued, as has been demonstrated by recent cases in Tanzania and Bolivia.

Rich countries: pushing the private sector, breaking aid promises, and taking teachers and nurses from poor countries

Rich country governments and international agencies such as the World Bank can have a major influence on policies adopted by poor countries. For some of the poorest countries, donor aid is equivalent to half the national budget. Advice from outside experts, funded by aid, is highly influential in determining the kinds of reforms a government adopts.

Instead of helping to build public services, rich country governments and agencies such as the World Bank too often use this influence to push private sector solutions to public service failures. They see the increased involvement of the private sector as the key to increasing efficiency and improving services, but growing evidence shows that these solutions rarely work in the interests of poor people. The World Bank and the IMF often insist that governments introduce privatisation and increase private service provision in return for aid or debt cancellation. A 2006 study of 20 countries receiving World Bank and IMF loans found that privatisation was a condition in 18 of them, an increase compared with previous years.

What poor country governments *need* is aid that is well co-ordinated, predictable, and channelled through public systems and national budgets. What poor countries typically *get* is insufficient, unpredictable aid, disbursed through a jumble of different projects that directly compete with public services for scarce resources and staff. As much as 70 per cent of aid for education globally is spent on technical assistance, much of it to highly paid Western consultants. A study of technical assistance in Mozambique found that rich countries were spending $350 million per year on technical experts, while the entire wage bill for Mozambique's public sector was just $74 million. In health, donor demands for numerous different 'vertical' initiatives waste officials' time, duplicate and undermine health delivery, and distort health priorities. Angola and the Democratic Republic of Congo, for instance, have each been required to set up four separate HIV/AIDS 'co-ordinating' bodies.

What poor country governments need is aid that is well co-ordinated, predictable, and channelled through public systems and national budgets.

IMF-imposed ceilings on public sector wages and recruitment prevent governments from expanding health and education services. While the IMF is right that countries should manage their economies carefully, its overly rigid stance is incompatible with achieving the Millennium Development Goals on health, education, and water and sanitation. The World Trade Organisation and bilateral and regional 'Free Trade Agreements' may also threaten public services by limiting how governments regulate foreign service providers.

At the same time as they are urging developing countries to meet the MDGs on health and education, rich countries are aggravating skills shortages by taking thousands of their key workers. Of the 489 students who graduated from the Ghana Medical School between 1986 and 1995, 61 per cent have left Ghana, with more than half of them going to the UK and one-third to the US.

What needs to happen

Change is possible, but it will take concerted action by developing country governments, supported, not undermined, by rich countries, and held to account by active citizens demanding their rights.

Shift the political agenda

Political commitment and the will to reform is key to making services work, and to do this governments must feel the heat. They must be pressured to spend more on essential services and to spend it better. In Kerala state in India and in Sri Lanka, politically-aware citizens demanded services that performed well. Across the world, civil society organisations are getting debates on essential services into the newspapers and onto politicians' lists of priorities. In Kenya the national coalition of education groups, Elimu Yetu (Our Education) played a pivotal role in making free primary education a central election issue, ensuring it was introduced in 2002; the result was that 1.2 million children went to school for the first time. In 2005 the world's biggest ever anti-poverty coalition was formed, the Global Call to Action against Poverty (GCAP). GCAP saw over 36 million people take action in more than 80 countries. Its key demands include quality universal public services for all and an end to privatisation where it causes deprivation and poverty.

Make services work for women

Investing in basic services that support and empower women and girls means promoting women as workers, supporting women and girls as service users, protecting them from abuse, and combining these measures with legal reforms that improve the status and autonomy of women in society. In Botswana, Mauritius, Sri Lanka, Costa Rica, and Cuba, the high proportion of women among teachers and health workers was instrumental in encouraging women and girls to use the services. Progress is often achieved by simultaneously working with women's groups, changing laws, and challenging harmful beliefs. In Brazil, women's organisations working within and outside government ensured that the 1988 Constitution reflected the importance of women's reproductive health. Women's movements have continued to influence public health policy in Brazil: an integrated women's health programme has been established (Programa de Assistencia a Saude da Mulher – PAISM) and special health services are now available to victims of rape.

Tackle the workforce crisis

> *'As long as there is breath in my body, I will continue to teach. I am not teaching because of the pay but because I love the job and I love children.'*
> Viola Shaw-Lewis, 76-year-old teacher, Kingsville public school, Liberia

Public sector workers must be seen for the heroes they are, and put at the heart of expanding services for all. All successful countries have built an ethos of public service, in which public sector workers are encouraged to take pride in their contribution to the nation, and society in turn is urged to grant them status and respect.

Pay on its own does not always increase motivation, but it is the first priority where earnings are currently too low. Better pay needs to be matched with better conditions. Housing is a major issue for most teachers, especially women teachers in rural areas. Governments must work with trade unions to achieve improved pay and conditions, combining them with codes of conduct to ensure that workers do their jobs.

Drastically scaling up the numbers of teachers and health workers is a huge task that requires strategic, co-ordinated planning between poor country governments and aid donors. Governments must invest in competent managers and planners to produce and implement clearly costed plans. In Malawi, donors are now funding a salary increase for public health workers, stemming the tide of doctors and nurses leaving for other countries and improving the quality of care on the wards.

Fight corruption and build accountability

In many cases, improved salaries, status, and conditions for public sector workers have helped to reduce small-scale corruption. At the level of society as a whole, strong public education services and public awareness campaigns can play an important role in promoting a culture of trust, honesty, and respect for the rule of law. Corruption also needs to be tackled at the political level. Multi-party democracy and the emergence of civil society and a free press are proving to be central in this fight. In Costa Rica and Kenya, for example, press scandals have led to the prosecution of senior officials for corruption.

Civil society is also playing an increasingly important and vocal role in holding political leaders to account, tracking government expenditures on essential services, and highlighting instances where money is going missing. Citizens need a formally recognised role in public oversight. WaterAid has set up feedback mechanisms between water user groups and local governments in Nepal, India, Bangladesh, Ghana, and Ethiopia. In Malawi education groups track government spending to the primary school level. The Social Watch international network unites citizens' groups in over 60 countries to regularly monitor the performance of their governments in the provision of essential services.

Public sector workers must be seen for the heroes they are, and put at the heart of expanding services for all.

Abolishing user fees for primary schooling and basic health care can have an immediate impact on the take-up of services.

Abolish user fees for primary education and basic health care

Abolishing user fees for primary schooling and basic health care can have an immediate impact on the take-up of services. For water, which no-one can do without, the issue is not take-up but improving access for poor people and ensuring that a finite resource is shared equitably. Fees must then be structured to ensure that a minimum daily amount is free or affordable for poor people.

Rich countries must support public services

Rich countries need to support developing country governments and peoples in implementing the kinds of measures outlined above. They must stop bypassing and undermining governments by pushing for the expansion of private service provision. They must meet their 36-year-old commitment to give 0.7 per cent of their income in foreign aid. This aid must be long-term, predictable, and targeted to countries that demonstrate their commitment to increase coverage of quality essential social services. It should be focused especially on providing salaries and the running costs for public systems, wherever possible through sectoral and direct budget support. This must further be supported by the full cancellation of debts for all the poor countries that need it. Rich governments must also reduce their active recruitment of professionals from poor countries to work in rich country health and education services.

Conclusion

Within a generation, for the first time in history, every child in the world could be in school. Every woman could give birth with the best possible chance that neither she nor her baby would die. Everyone could drink water without risking their lives. Millions of new health workers and teachers could be saving lives and shaping minds.

We know how to get there: political leadership, government action, and public services, supported by long-term flexible aid from rich countries and the cancellation of debt. We know that the market alone cannot do this. Civil society can pick up some of the pieces, but governments must act. There is no short cut, and no other way.

To achieve these goals, developing country governments must fulfil their responsibilities, their citizens must pressure them to do so, and rich countries must support and not undermine them. In the words of Nelson Mandela:

> *'Poverty is not natural. It is man-made and it can be overcome and eradicated by the actions of human beings. And overcoming poverty is not a gesture of charity. It is an act of justice. It is the protection of a fundamental human right; the right to dignity and a decent life. While poverty persists, there is no freedom.'*
> Speech at launch of Make Poverty History campaign, Trafalgar Square, London, 3 February 2005

Recommendations

Developing country governments need to:

- Make sustained investments in essential education, health care, and water and sanitation systems and services. Specifically, they must emphasise preventative reproductive health policies and actively combat the HIV/AIDS pandemic.
- Abolish fees for basic education and health care and subsidise water for poor people.
- Enhance equity by making services work for women and girls and by improving their social status.
- Work with civil society and the private sector within a single, integrated public system.
- Train, recruit, and retain desperately needed health workers and teachers.
- Improve the pay and conditions of existing workers.
- Build an ethos of public service, in which both the public and essential service workers are encouraged to take pride in their contribution.
- Ensure citizen representation and oversight in monitoring public services and facilitate the participation of civil society in local and national planning and budget processes, including agreements and contracts signed with donors, the World Bank, and the IMF.
- Take a public stand and act against corruption.

Rich countries, the World Bank, and the IMF need to:

- Halt the pursuit of inappropriate market reforms of public services through aid conditions, technical advice, and trade agreements.
- Keep their promise to give 0.7 per cent of their national income as foreign aid and to allocate at least 20 per cent of that aid to basic services.
- Fully implement international commitments to improve aid quality, including the Paris commitments on aid effectiveness. Ensure that such aid is co-ordinated, predictable, and long-term, including further debt cancellation and increased budget and sector support.
- Financially support the removal of user fees in basic health care and education and the subsidising of water fees for poor people.
- Fully finance the Global Fund to Fight AIDS, TB and Malaria, and the Education for All Fast Track Initiative, ensuring that they support governments and public systems, rather than duplicating their activities.
- Work with poor countries to recruit, train, and retain 4.25 million new health workers and 1.9 million teachers, and invest in the skills of public utility and local government staff responsible for delivering water and sanitation services.
- Reduce the active recruitment of health and other professionals from poor countries.

- Act together to demand quality public services, including free health care and education and subsidised water and sanitation services.

- Continue to build worldwide popular movements demanding government action, such as the Global Campaign for Education, the Global Call to Action against Poverty, and the women's movement.

- Engage in local and national planning processes.

- Work with national parliaments to monitor budget spending, to ensure that services are reaching the poorest people, and that corruption is not tolerated.

- Challenge rich country governments, the World Bank, and the IMF when they fail to support public services.

- Work closely with government and other non-state providers to ensure increased innovation, learning, co-operation, and accountability in the provision of essential services.

1
Essential services:
failing to meet essential needs

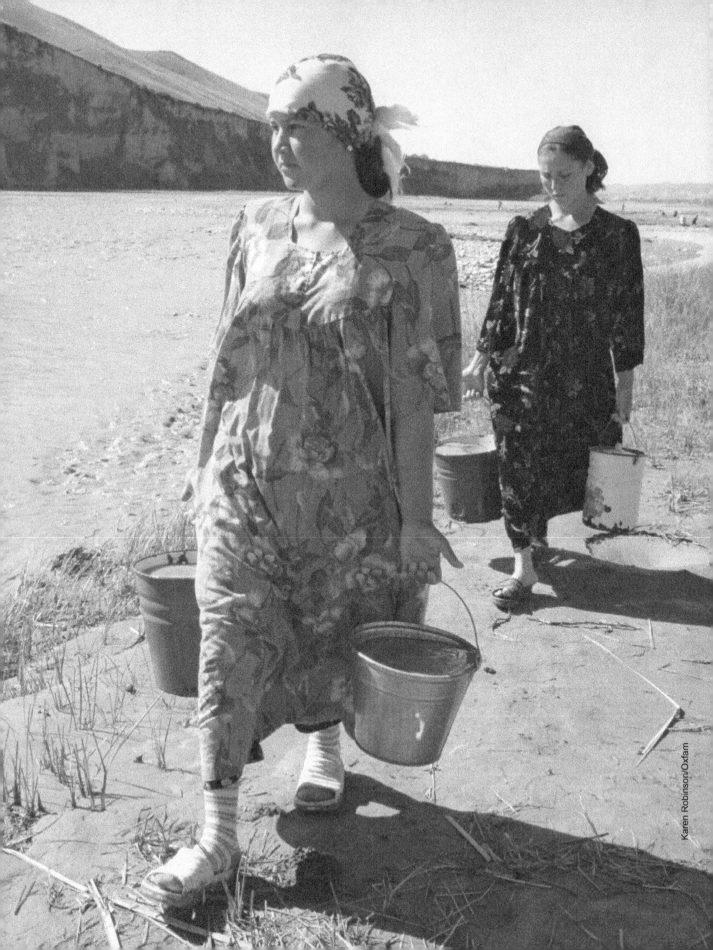

1
Essential services: failing to meet essential needs

'We manage to impart lessons [by] the skin of our teeth, because we get no resources from the Ministry of Education. We no longer get the materials we used to, such as notebooks and pencils or chalk, or textbooks for the children.'
Head teacher, Jose Madriz Autonomous School, Nicaragua

'I will never forget how I suffered due to the lack of water. There was no water to wash the baby or myself. I was ashamed of the unpleasant smell, especially when my neighbours visited me.'
Misra Kedir, recalling her child's birth, Hitosa, Ethiopia

Classrooms with teachers. Clinics with nurses. Running taps and working toilets. Essential services transform people's lives. It is a scandal that anyone lives without them in 2006. Yet millions of families do. The lack of essential services sets the poverty trap: people cannot escape poverty when they cannot read or write, are wasted by ill health, or have to spend hours a day fetching water.

If ever there was a time to fulfil these most basic of human rights — decent health care, education, and water and sanitation for all — then this is it. These rights are enshrined in international covenants[1] and have been assigned targets by the international community. The Millennium Development Goals commit governments by 2015 to:

- Eradicate extreme poverty and hunger, and to halve the proportion of people living on less than one dollar per day and the proportion of people who suffer from hunger.
- Achieve universal primary education (UPE) for boys and girls.
- Promote gender equality and empower women by eliminating gender disparity in primary and secondary education by 2005, and at all levels of education by 2015.
- Reduce child mortality by cutting the under-five mortality rate by two-thirds.
- Improve maternal health, and reduce by three-quarters the maternal mortality ratio.
- Combat HIV/AIDS, malaria, and other diseases, and reverse the spread of HIV/AIDS.
- Ensure environmental sustainability, halve the proportion of people without access to potable water, and improve the lives of 100 million slum dwellers.
- Develop a global partnership for development, raise the volume of aid, and improve market access.

opposite page
Collecting water in Shibanai village, Tajikistan. Saodat and Osuda Hasanova fetch water two or three times every day: *'It's really hard work because the water buckets are so heavy... I've heard that in other places people just turn on a tap in their house and the water comes out. I would love a tap like that in our house*

The world can certainly afford to act. Oxfam calculates that meeting the Millennium Development Goal targets on health, education, and water and sanitation would require an extra $47 billion a year.[2] Compare this with annual global military spending of $1 trillion, or the $40 billion that the world spends every year on pet food.[3] But with 'development as usual', most of these targets will be missed. 2005 has already come and gone, and with it the first target of equalising education between girls and boys, missed in two out of every three developing countries.[4]

Governments have a clear duty to meet these targets and to guarantee the welfare of their citizens. People have rights to decent health care, to learn to read and write, to have safe water to drink, and to the sanitary disposal of human waste. But in too many countries governments fail because of a lack of cash, a lack of capacity, or a lack of commitment. Too often, rich country governments have contributed to this problem by failing to make good their financial promises to poor countries, or by pushing market-based reforms that unravel public systems, and public responsibilities, still further.

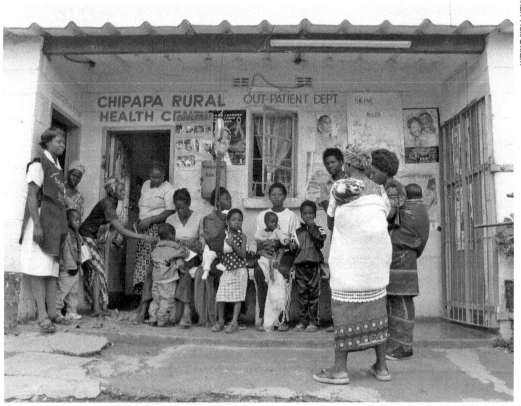

Jonah Hull/Oxfam

Chipapa Health clinic, Zambia
Investing in girls and women is the cornerstone of human development.

The most glaring failure has been in making services work for women and girls. A decent level of welfare is the first step in improving women's well-being and status in society. Investing in women and girls is also the cornerstone of human development: sending a girl to school and caring for her basic health reduces the number of children she is likely to have over her lifetime, increases the chances that she and her infant will survive childbirth, and improves the prospects of her children as they grow. It also enhances her household's ability to earn income, and deepens her own participation in political life. Few investments offer such rich returns.

Despite all this — and despite so many declarations and international conferences over the years — essential services are still failing women and, through them, society. Across the developing world, women are more likely than men to fall ill, but less likely to receive medical care. They are expected to be 'available, prepared, and morally obliged'[5] to care for other family members when they fall ill. Girls are too often the last in the family to be sent to school and the first to be taken out when money is short, or else they cannot go to school because there is no girls' latrine. And it is — almost always, everywhere — girls and women who lose so much of their day to hauling buckets of water over long distances.

Across the developing world, women are more likely than men to fall ill, but less likely to receive medical care.

This widespread failure to deliver decent essential services, and to make them serve women and girls, as well as men and boys, is fundamentally undermining the prospects of achieving the Millennium Development Goals (see Figure 1).

Figure 1: Missing the target: global progress towards the MDGs

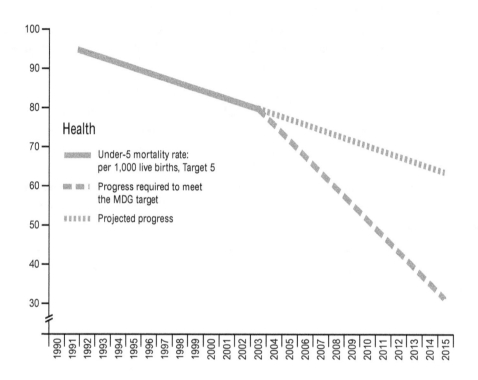

Health

- Under-5 mortality rate: per 1,000 live births, Target 5
- Progress required to meet the MDG target
- Projected progress

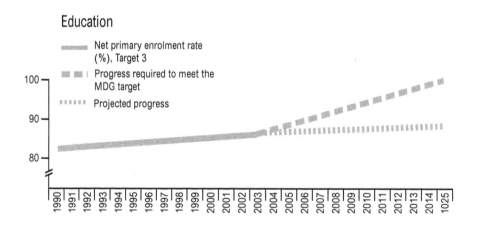

Education

- Net primary enrolment rate (%), Target 3
- Progress required to meet the MDG target
- Projected progress

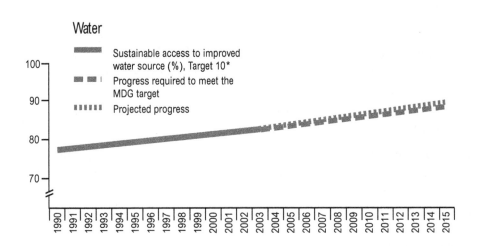

Water

- Sustainable access to improved water source (%), Target 10*
- Progress required to meet the MDG target
- Projected progress

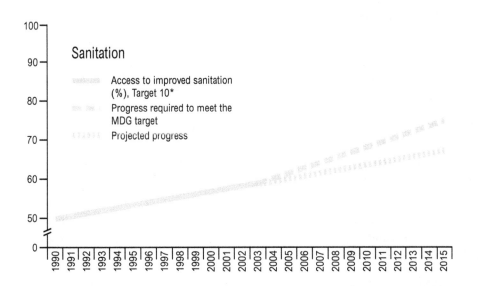

Sanitation

- Access to improved sanitation (%), Target 10*
- Progress required to meet the MDG target
- Projected progress

(Source: United Nations Statistics Division, http://unstats.un.org/unsd/mi/mi_worldregn.asp)
* Water sources and sanitation are deemed as 'improved' according to a list of criteria set by the United Nations
(e.g. whether there is a household water connection or pit latrine).

Water and sanitation: far off-track

International commitments to the MDG targets lose any credibility when measured against the current provision of water and sanitation facilities around the world. In most regions the international target to halve the proportion of people who have no clean drinking water is far off-track and, in total, will fail 210 million people.[6] On current progress, Africa will not meet the goal until the year 2105. One in three people in the world does not have access to any kind of toilet or latrine and, contrary to international promises, this number is increasing.[7] Today more than one billion people still live without clean water.[8]

More than one billion people still live without clean water.

Water-related diseases cause three million deaths a year[9] and the worst impacts fall on young children: diarrhoea, a disease of dirty water, is the biggest killer of under-fives in poor countries, resulting in 4,000 preventable deaths every day.[10] The lives of women and girls are badly affected by the lack of safe water and latrines: many walk up to four miles a day to fetch water,[11] or wait till dusk or dawn to relieve themselves in the fields or bush, where they risk sexual harassment.

Meeting the MDG target to halve the number of people without access to clean water would cost $4 billion a year for ten years — roughly a month's spending on bottled mineral water in Europe or the USA.[12] It could save money too: for every $1 invested, another $3–$4 is saved on health spending or through increased productivity.[13] Failing to provide water and sanitation will cost developing countries $84 billion per year in lost lives, low worker productivity, higher health-care costs, and lost education opportunities.[14]

Health: enduring inequalities

The past ten years have seen slow and piecemeal progress towards the agreed health targets. Yet simple, low-cost technologies could save the lives of the 11 million children who die each year from preventable communicable diseases such as measles and diarrhoea, and from malnutrition.[15]

Meanwhile, HIV/AIDS has inflicted an unprecedented reversal in human development — 40 million people are now infected with the disease. HIV/AIDS claimed 3 million lives in 2005, orphaning millions of children,[16] and is leaving health systems struggling to cope, with women increasingly shouldering the burden. In sub-Saharan Africa, 57 per cent of adults living with HIV/AIDS are women,[17] while young women account for a disproportionate number of new HIV infections. In some settings, being married may actually increase women's exposure to the disease — in Thailand, 75 per cent of women infected with HIV/AIDS were probably infected by their husbands.[18]

There has been some progress: in 1990, only 41 per cent of women giving birth in developing countries were attended by a trained nurse or midwife; by 2003 that proportion had risen to

57 per cent[19] — although none of this progress was to the benefit of new mothers in sub-Saharan Africa. However, bad news outweighs the good. Women in developing countries still have a one in 61 chance of dying from a pregnancy-related cause: compare that with one in 2,800 in developed countries.[20]

Education: signs of progress

If there is any cause for hope regarding essential services, it is the progress made in the past 15 years in getting young children into school. Every region (with the exception of the former Soviet Union) has significantly increased primary school enrolments, particularly Latin America, the Caribbean, and North Africa.[21] Enrolments in sub-Saharan Africa have grown fast too. Even some of Africa's poorest countries — Eritrea, Guinea, Malawi, and Chad — have increased primary enrolments by over 50 per cent, albeit from a very low base.[22]

International momentum has been crucial in achieving these results. The right to universal and free primary education, enshrined in declarations for many decades,[23] was finally recognised as a reality through an agreed global vision of how to get all children into school: the Education For All framework.[24] This was backed up by some — but by no means all — of the funding needed to achieve it, mobilised both by means of poor country governments giving it higher priority in their national budgets, and by rich country aid donors co-ordinating their aid more effectively through the Fast Track Initiative.[25] Campaigning by many civil society coalitions across the world was essential to ensure that those plans and funds were turned into universal and free education for children.

Enormous challenges remain. Some 100 million children are still out of school — 18 per cent of the world's primary school-age population[26] — and the MDG target of universal primary education will be missed on current trends. Many of these missing students are girls living in rural areas, who are required to work in the fields or help in the home, or who suddenly find themselves heading the household after their parents have died from AIDS. Some are children from indigenous or ethnic minority communities who may not understand the language used in the classroom. Others may have a disability that the school is unable to accommodate. All of them have the right to an education, and hence to the policies that will make this possible for them.

Some 100 million children are still out of school — 18 per cent of the world's primary school-age population.

Yet even in countries where most children have started going to school, governments are often failing to keep them there. Completion rates — i.e. the proportion of school-age children who complete the final year of primary school — are depressingly low in many countries. Only half of all boys, and even fewer girls, complete primary school in sub-Saharan Africa. As a result, the average 16-year-old girl in Africa has had less than three years of schooling.[27]

Often the reason is the low quality of the education on offer. Many schools lack sufficient textbooks and teachers to cater for their many pupils, or use a curriculum that has little relevance to the needs of local communities. Too many dispirited teachers rely on teaching by rote, instead of engaging children in active learning. Female students often report feeling intimidated or disrespected by the classroom culture. Such learning environments do not provide girls or boys with the skills they need in adult life, and offer little incentive to children who have to walk for hours each day just to get to school. Enrolments and achievements will clearly only be raised, and sustained, by raising the quality of education systems.

The strides made in primary enrolments show that progress is possible, when the political commitment is backed by national and international financing. But what works, and why isn't everyone doing it?

2
What works?
The case for universal public services

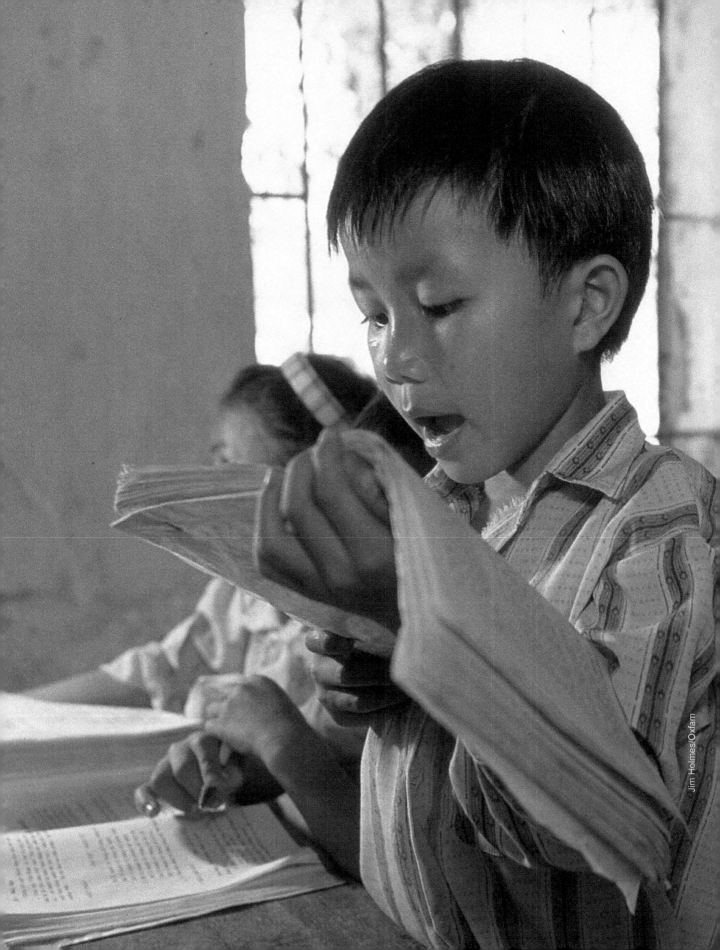

2
What works? The case for universal public services

'My son had a temperature and diarrhoea. He kept throwing up but at La Mascota they didn't want to help him, they turned me away. So I came straight here and the doctor immediately admitted him, otherwise the child would have died. Here we don't have to pay. This is a public hospital specially for children and pregnant women.'
Julisa Ramirez, Fernando Velez Paiz Maternity Hospital, Nicaragua

'The provision of basic education, the presence of elementary medical facilities, the availability of resources [such as water]... these non-market facilities require careful and determined public action.'
Amartya Sen, *Development as Freedom*

More than one-third of Sri Lanka's population live on less than two dollars a day, but the country's maternal mortality rates are among the lowest in the world. Over the course of the 1990s the number of maternal deaths halved, from 520 to 250 women per year, in a population of 18 million. Today over 96 per cent of deliveries are attended by a skilled birth attendant and over 90 per cent take place in a health facility. How has this been achieved? By providing public health services free of charge — essential in making them accessible to poor people — and by providing a large number of health posts: almost everyone now lives less than 1.5km from their nearest centre. These measures have been strongly supported by education policies that provide free education for girls up to university level, resulting in a literacy rate of 88 per cent among adult women and an increase in the average age of marriage.[28]

Incomes matter, but policies matter too

Many other countries — including poor ones — have made huge strides in human welfare. To try and assess government performance in providing essential services, Oxfam has devised an Essential Services Index. This ranks countries according to their performance in four social areas — child survival rates, schooling, access to safe water, and access to sanitation — and compares their performance with per capita national income.[29] The comparison shows that

opposite page
Hoang Zuan (seven) reading aloud during a language lesson in Ky Hai primary school, Viet Nam

some governments have consistently punched above their weights. Sri Lanka, for example, has 60 per cent less income per capita than Kazakhstan ($4,000 a year compared with $6,980), but a child in Kazakhstan is nearly five times more likely to die in its first five years than a child in Sri Lanka and is far less likely to go to school, drink clean water, or have the use of a latrine (see Figure 2).

Figure 2: Sri Lanka: less income than Kazakhstan, but healthier, better-educated people

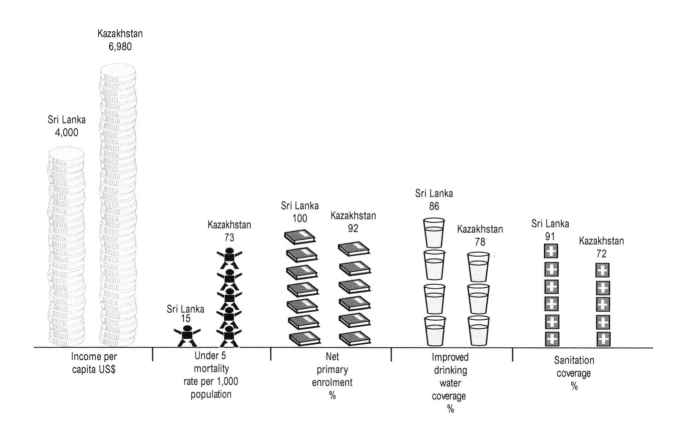

(Source: Essential Services Index, data compiled by Oxfam)

These discrepancies in performance relative to income occur at all levels of income. As Figure 3 shows, countries such as Sri Lanka, the Philippines, Uganda, and Bangladesh all perform above their expected level, while countries such as Brazil, Oman, and Mauritania are all delivering far lower welfare outcomes than would be expected, given their per capita incomes. Wealth matters, but so does government action.

Figure 3: Higher income levels do not always determine outcomes

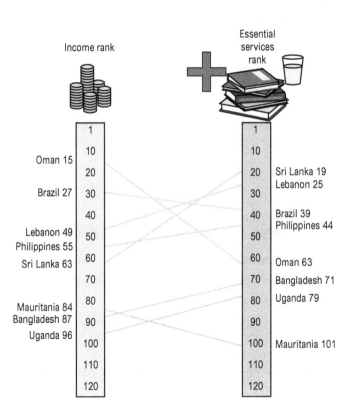

(Source: Essential Services Index, data compiled by Oxfam)

Economic growth does not determine performance either — although it is certainly necessary in the long term. Successful countries did not wait until they became rich to invest in essential services. Indeed, the East Asian 'tiger' economies are renowned for investing in essential services *before* their economic take-offs.

When governments get it right: learning from success

The next decade must see a massive scaling up in the provision of essential services if the Millennium Development Goals are to be met. Millions more teachers and health workers are needed in hundreds of thousands more schools and clinics worldwide, along with engineers and sewerage systems, boreholes, taps, and toilets.

The pivotal question is how best to achieve this expansion. To answer this question we need to look at the experience of countries — both developed and developing — that have succeeded in scaling up essential services. What this section will show is that the key to success is action by governments in funding, co-ordinating, and providing these essential services to the public. Governments have to act, because the provision of services by the market alone will not provide for poor people.

The case for government action

There are strong economic and social reasons why governments need to organise essential services, rather than leaving it up to individuals or to pay for them through the market.[30]

Firstly, if people are healthy and well-educated, it benefits the economic and social well-being of the population as a whole, over and above the health and economic status of each individual. Curing a person of a communicable disease such as tuberculosis benefits not just that individual, but everyone who may otherwise have caught the disease. Increasing the level of girls' education will bring positive benefits to the next generation of children. Markets and price mechanisms do not reflect the true value of such 'public goods', since they encourage individuals to pay only for benefits to themselves, not to society as a whole.

Secondly, citizens do not always have the full information necessary to make informed choices about the services they need, or who should provide them. This is a particularly important issue in health care, where it is easy for a provider to mislead patients into buying care that is inappropriate or unneeded. Government action is required to inform people of the benefits of healthy behaviour, even on such a simple level as hand-washing.

Thirdly, people in poor countries, particularly in rural areas, seldom have a choice of provider, whether of schools, clinics, or water supply. In fact they are often lucky to have any of these services at all. This means that competition, the main engine for efficiency in a market, is absent. Governments generally have access to cheaper forms of credit than those available to the private sector, which makes large capital investments, such as infrastructure for urban sanitation, easier to finance.

Leaving essential services such as education to the market increases inequality, as poor people are less able to pay for services. Since education is strongly linked to future incomes, these inequalities are passed down through the generations, as poor families find themselves unable to give their children a decent, healthy start in life.

Finally, access to good quality essential services is a human right that should not be denied to people simply because they are unable to pay for them. Governments are the duty bearers and have a responsibility to deliver on people's human rights.

These arguments show that public action is necessary to organise essential services, but do not explain who should provide them. However, as the next section shows, both historical and current experience demonstrate that public provision is key to essential services.

Government action was the key to advances in developed nations

During the nineteenth century, governments in rich countries stepped in to develop public services.[31] In the UK the inefficiencies, costs, and corruption of private sector water provision led to the creation of public water and sanitation systems.[32] In Germany the national health system unified multiple insurance schemes under one equitable system. Compulsory public education was extended across Europe, North America, and Japan in the early part of the century and these welfare states expanded further after World War Two.

At the dawn of the twentieth century the UK was the world's leading industrial nation, yet its average life expectancy then was at a level that is common in Africa today. Extensive public programmes, particularly in sanitation, but also in health and nutrition, were the key to a rapidly rising life expectancy during the course of the century.

The impact of government *inaction* is clear in the United States, the only wealthy nation today with no universal health insurance system. Its mix of private employer-based insurance and limited public health care is linked to extreme inequalities in health outcomes, leaving over one-third of people living below the poverty line in 2003 without health insurance. The Institute of Medicine[33] estimates that 18,000 Americans die prematurely each year because they lack health insurance. Such a system is also inefficient: the USA spends more as a proportion of GDP on health care than any other nation, but has a higher infant mortality rate than many other industrialised countries.[34]

At the dawn of the twentieth century the UK was the world's leading industrial nation, yet its average life expectancy then was at a level that is common in Africa today. Extensive public programmes were the key to a rapidly rising life expectancy during the course of the century.

Government action has also underpinned success in developing countries

In recent decades, many developing countries have achieved extraordinary progress. Within a generation, they have made advances in health and education that took industrialised countries 200 years to accomplish. In various 'breakthrough' periods Botswana, Zimbabwe, Mauritius, Sri Lanka, South Korea, Malaysia, Barbados, Costa Rica, Cuba, and Kerala state in India[35] all cut child deaths by between 40 per cent and 70 per cent in just 10 years.[36] All also achieved primary school enrolments close to 100 per cent for both girls and boys, decades before other developing countries.[37] In Zimbabwe these advances have since been undermined by economic and political crisis, and in Botswana by the ravages of HIV/AIDS, but their examples still show that rapid progress can be made by poor countries.

Before the collapse of the Soviet Union, public services such as free health care greatly increased the quality of life, particularly in the poorest Central Asian republics.[38] In East Asian countries, the importance of the links between equitable access to social provision, poverty reduction, and growth was recognised early on. The Indonesian government, for example, massively expanded public education in the 1970s and now runs 150,000 primary schools, covering 85 per cent of all enrolments.[39]

In the early 1980s Nicaragua raised adult literacy rates from 47 per cent to 87 per cent and increased access to health care from 25 per cent to 70 per cent of the population, as part of a major programme of public investment following the Sandinista revolution.[40] Similarly, in 1982 a World Health Organization survey of Mozambican health services found that the massive expansion of rural public health posts overseen by the Frelimo government meant that 81 per cent of children had been seen by a health worker (24 years later, this is still an amazing achievement in Africa).

Lessons from developing country success

The critical factor has been concerted action by governments in organising and providing public services for all.

Studies of the policies underpinning developing country success stories show that, despite some differences in approach, the measures taken by successful countries have much in common.[41] The critical factor has been concerted action by governments in organising and providing public services for all. This has been the case regardless of whether the state in question was socialist Cuba or capitalist South Korea.[42] Governments built universal essential services, which were paid for through progressive taxation and prioritised spending, and delivered through strong public systems, free or heavily subsidised for poor people — and all geared to the needs of women and girls.

Clear political commitment and pressure from civil society

Those developing countries that have succeeded have all had high-level political commitment from their ruling elites and middle classes to improving the general welfare of their citizens, and especially that of poor people. Fighting poverty became a political issue. The people of Barbados, for instance, started calling for social progress in the 1930s; health and education services have been a feature of political party competition since multi-party elections began in the 1950s. In Nicaragua and Mozambique, the expansion of public services formed a key part of the countries' revolutions and struggles for independence. The reasons for middle-class and elite commitment varied, from the moral and ideological to enlightened self-interest. However, extensive mobilisation by citizens demanding their rights was a common thread in many of the success stories, as leaders sought to respond to the demands of their people.

Universally accessible, publicly provided

In countries successful at providing essential services, the vast majority of the population used services provided by the state, with just the wealthiest opting for private health care and schooling. Primary education was state-provided and health services were universal, not targeted, and funded from government revenues.[43] These policies made good economic sense (and still do today) in countries where poverty was so widespread that poor people constituted the majority of the population.

In countries successful at providing essential services, the vast majority of the population used services provided by the state.

In many countries, improving services has meant consolidating a fragmented mix of public, private, and non-profit health and education providers. Typically, successful governments have sought to integrate non-state providers (NSPs) into public delivery systems to complement public systems, rather than as a substitute for them. In Kerala state, Malaysia, and Barbados, governments funded the running costs of private schools and church schools and regularly inspected and monitored them to maintain standards.[44]

Free at the point of delivery

> '*I think we have many good things in our country. The schools are totally free; education in Cuba is both free and good. We pay absolutely nothing.*'
> Leonor Diaz, mother of schoolchild, Cuba

Abolishing user fees for health and education resulted in massive increases in school enrolments and the uptake of health services in all countries. For newly independent countries this was also a political statement, signalling that access to essential services was a basic human right. The introduction of free education in Tanzania and many other African nations in the 1960s was an important part of defining the rights of citizens, following independence from colonial rule. Similarly, in the majority of countries, there were low or no out-of-pocket costs for poor people using health services.

Teacher Richard Machibya
and his Standard 2
maths class,
Shinyanga, Tanzania

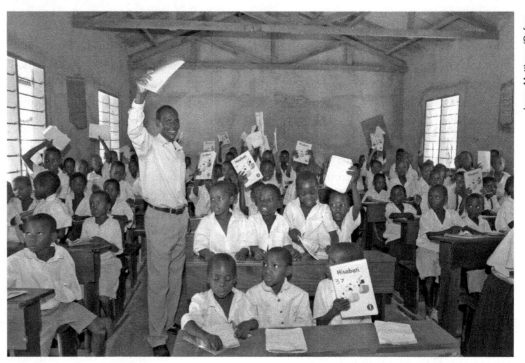

Jenny Matthews/Oxfam

*In low-income countries,
the most pro-poor
health systems were
those providing
universal services
that were free or
almost free.*

A UK government-funded study comparing health systems across Asia[45] found that in low-income countries, the most pro-poor health systems were those providing universal services that were free or almost free. When fees were reintroduced in Zimbabwe under structural adjustment, the effect on poor people's access to services was catastrophic. In some countries there were additional subsidies to reduce the cost of services for households, such as free school meals in Kerala, Sri Lanka, Zimbabwe, Barbados, Costa Rica, and Cuba.

Water and sanitation: affordable and available

Successful countries make providing safe water and sanitation a priority.[46] In Costa Rica, for example, water supply, latrine construction, and public education on hygienic practices went hand-in-hand with extending rural health services. The government of Botswana invested in a major programme of groundwater drilling and water network construction soon after independence in 1966, achieving near-universal access to safe water by the 1990s. Rural households were subsidised to build latrines and the government invested in health and hygiene education programmes.

Investing in teachers and nurses, and serving rural areas

Massive increases in human resources have been at the heart of the successful provision of public services in poor countries. Successful countries invested heavily in training and in employing front-line workers — teachers, health workers, and water technicians. Brazil still has a long way to go to improve child health, but had increased net school enrolment rates to near 100 per cent for girls and boys by 1997, by instituting broad-based national reforms to improve teacher qualifications and training, along with performance-related pay and increased salaries with generous pension benefits.[47] Uganda's near doubling of net enrolments, from 54 per cent to over 90 per cent by 2000, was preceded by fundamental reforms, including an increase in teachers' salaries from $8 to $72 per month from 1997.[48]

Governments also ensured that rural facilities were well staffed, often by requiring publicly trained workers to work in rural areas. In Sri Lanka, all teachers are expected to work for 3–4 years in 'difficult schools', and a teacher deployment project has implemented a 'staff equalisation plan' that penalises provinces with excessive numbers of teachers and provides resources for provinces with teacher shortages.[49] In the Gambia the government is building new housing in remote areas and establishing a 'teacher housing loan scheme' to help female teachers with the costs of decent accommodation.[50]

Nicaragua, China, Zimbabwe, and Cuba trained thousands of village health workers and 'barefoot doctors' to provide preventative health care and hygiene education. In Nicaragua thousands of volunteers helped in a hugely successful national literacy campaign. In Zimbabwe housing was supplied for rural health workers, which sharply reduced the number of rural vacancies in essential services. Kerala and Sri Lanka relied heavily on recruiting and employing midwives within their own communities.

Building long-term public capacity to deliver

All successful countries invested heavily in building infrastructure and improving public capacity to plan, deliver, and co-ordinate reforms. Public spending prioritised essential services as governments pursued progressive taxation, mobilising resources from the richest sections of society to spend on services for the poorest. Health and education spending[51] were higher than the regional averages for all successful countries (except in South Korea). Social programmes took priority in government budgets: in Costa Rica such programmes commanded some 50 per cent of the budget, and in Kerala health and education spending accounted for around 40 per cent of the state budget. Primary services got priority: primary education, for example, received between a quarter and half of total education spending.

Uganda's near doubling of net enrolments was preceded by fundamental reforms, including an increase in teachers' salaries from $8 to $72 per month.

Improving services in high-performing countries required a massive expansion of publicly-funded infrastructure, especially in rural areas. Botswana and Mauritius, for example, both inherited tiny hospital-based health services at independence, but public construction and training programmes doubled the number of health posts so that, by the 1980s, at least 80 per cent of their populations lived within 15km of a health facility.

This investment was backed up by international aid. Virtually all roads, schools, and health facilities built in Botswana during the 1960s and 1970s were financed largely from donor sources, as part of a co-ordinated national development plan. Costa Rica received $3.4bn between 1970 and 1992, mostly from the USA, and this helped it to shield its social spending during the economic crisis of the 1980s. South Korea and Cuba benefited from direct foreign aid from the USA and the Soviet Union respectively; this was not always invested directly in health and education, but it helped to free up resources for essential services from other budget lines. Importantly, this aid did not undermine the ability of the recipient countries to make their own decisions on the best way to provide public services.

Investing in women makes services more effective and society more equal

The provision of public services in successful countries has made society more equitable, by focusing on women and girls. Governments have pursued gender equity in both the educational levels attained and in employment status: in Botswana, Zimbabwe, Mauritius, Sri Lanka, South Korea, Malaysia, Barbados, Costa Rica, Cuba, and Kerala state in India, women's and girls' access to education was higher than the regional average and there was a high proportion of female teachers and health workers, which encouraged others to use the services. This was all underpinned by government action to strengthen women's social status and autonomy — in Mauritius, Cuba, and South Africa new legislation enshrined the rights of women to own and inherit property, and their rights to freedom from violence and discrimination.

Special efforts to reach poor people

The Kerala state government in India expanded health-care facilities and ensured that over half its hospital beds were in rural hospitals and clinics.

Successful countries made particular efforts to reach poor people by expanding community-level primary services in rural areas. In all of them, primary school teaching was carried out in the local mother tongue to make learning easier. Costa Rica established community health programmes to immunise children, distributed milk, built latrines, and used geographical targeting criteria to prioritise the construction of health centres in poor areas. The Kerala state government in India expanded health-care facilities in the deprived Malabar region to reduce the inequality of health care between regions, and ensured that over half its hospital beds were in rural hospitals and clinics. Malaysia set up a three-tier scheme consisting of health centres, sub-centres, and midwife clinics to provide health services directly to the rural population.

Recent success stories have similar ingredients

More recent advances in services show a similar recipe to that of the success stories discussed above. Success has been built on strong public systems that guarantee universal access to free health care and education and subsidised water and sanitation for poor people, and on making services work for women and girls.

Uganda: extending access to schools and clinics

Uganda's primary school enrolments nearly doubled in a decade, from 54 per cent in 1991 to over 90 per cent by 2000.[52] Gender gaps in enrolments have been virtually eliminated: a stunning accomplishment for a low-income country emerging from civil war.

How did it happen? In 1997 the government introduced free schooling for up to four children in every household, increased teachers' salaries, integrated gender concerns into the national curriculum, and encouraged schools to buy new and better textbooks. How was it financed? By cutting the defence budget, and increasing education funds by almost 50 per cent.[53]

Throughout the 1990s, Ugandans faced high costs for fragmented health services. But in the run-up to the 2001 presidential election, President Yoweri Museveni ended user fees for all government health clinics. The public response was phenomenal, with an 84 per cent increase in attendance at clinics countrywide.[54] Mission hospitals were also brought into the public system and strengthened with public funds. The benefits were greatest for poor people in rural areas who could not afford to pay for care.[55]

Brazil: increasing access to clean water and providing free treatment for HIV/AIDS

Brazil still has a long way to go to address huge inequalities in access to services, but some government initiatives are beginning to make a difference. In 1994 the World Bank predicted that there would be 1.2 million HIV-positive Brazilians by 2000.[56] Six years later, the prevalence of the disease was only half that level, thanks to prompt government action. In 1996, the Brazilian government made antiretroviral treatment (ART) free for all those who needed it.[57] By 2005, 160,000 Brazilians were receiving ART, the annual death rate from AIDS had more than halved, and hospitalisation rates had fallen by over 75 per cent. The annual budget for the programme is $395m, but it has saved more than $2bn in public health costs since the epidemic started.[58]

By 2005, 160,000 Brazilians were receiving ART, the annual death rate from AIDS had more than halved, and hospitalisation rates had fallen by over 75 per cent.

The lowest infant mortality rate in Brazil is in the city of Porto Alegre, which is far from being the richest city. In a country of huge inequalities, how did this happen? Largely because the city's Municipal Department for Water and Sewage supplies clean water to 99.5 per cent of households at one of the cheapest rates in the country, and treats 84 per cent of its sewage. Up to 70 per cent of the operation is outsourced to private contractors, who collect payments through household water meters. Their contracts with the municipality ensure social equity: poor people have the right to use 10,000 litres of water per month, but only pay for 4,000.[59]

Sanitation in India and safe water in Malaysia

Sanitation in India has improved in recent years, thanks to the government's Total Sanitation Campaign, which aims to end the practice of open defecation by 2010.[60] The programme is succeeding by setting up production units to make latrines, giving incentives to poor households to build them, and providing hygiene education in schools.

In the Malaysian state of Pulau Penang, the public water utility, PBAPP, is highly efficient, supplying water to 100 per cent of urban residents and 99 per cent in rural areas (4 million people in total). And it is equitable: it sets a subsidised price for the first 20,000 litres of water used by a household each month, giving poorer consumers affordable access to drinking water. PBAPP is a public limited company owned by the government, and it strives to combine commercial efficiency with social objectives.[61] It has a workforce that is committed to excellence in public service and has achieved an international quality standard for its approach to quality management, its customer focus, and environmentally sustainable development.

Conclusion

The experiences of successful countries offer hope and inspiration for the future. They show that it is possible to achieve rapid and sustained gains in human welfare for poor people, even when a country is in the early stages of development. They also demonstrate that the key to this success is strong public systems that guarantee universal access to free health care and education and subsidised water and sanitation for poor people, and which make services work for women and girls. In most successful countries, states are the main provider of services. Even when there is a large degree of provision by the private sector, this works only when there are strong co-ordination, financing, and regulation by governments. It takes time to create the institutions, staff, and infrastructure to provide universal essential services, but with adequate and predictable finance, political will, and technical support, even the poorest countries can achieve this vital goal.

3

When it goes wrong:

poor country government neglect and broken promises

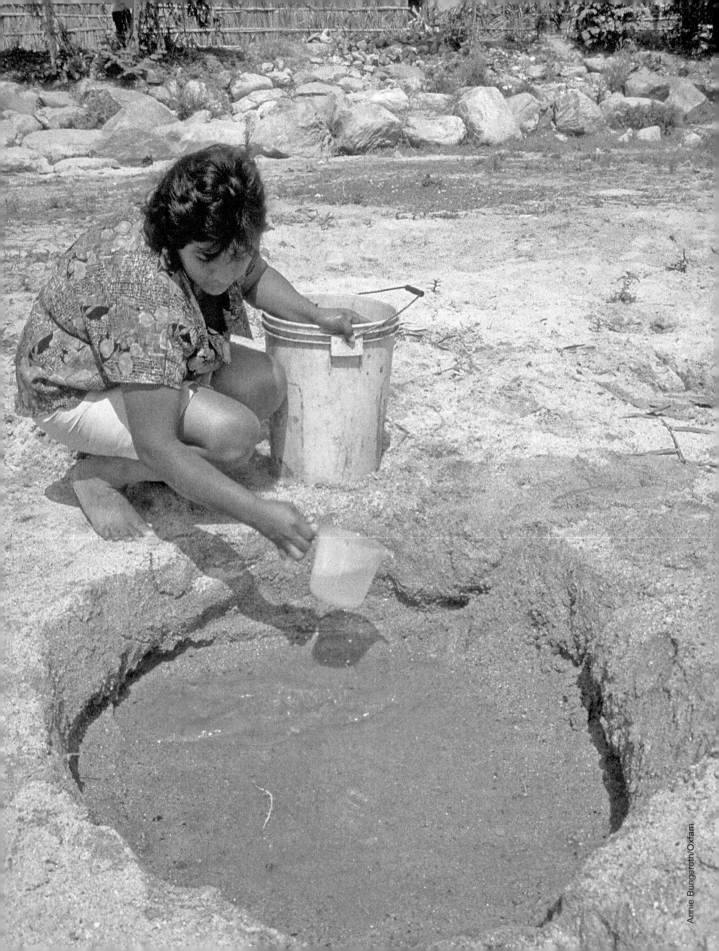

3
When it goes wrong: poor country government neglect and broken promises

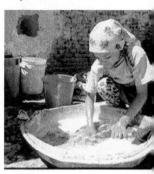

'We have to cross three creeks to reach our schools. These creeks swell up to four feet during rainy periods. When the rains come, our mother fears for our lives.' [62]
Primary schoolchildren in Kimarayag, Philippines

'In the health centre they get annoyed when they treat you. If you don't have any money they won't take you. If you don't have money, then what? Well, you'll just be left to die.'
Marta Maria Molina Aguilar, mother of sick child, Nicaragua

'After paying for electricity and water and buying food, there's nothing left. I can't survive on my salary. So I do shifts as a locum in a private hospital in Lilongwe. It's not good though. Our ways of surviving are killing the system.'
Dr. Matias Joshua, Dowa District Hospital, Malawi

Fatima from Al Samsarah, Yemen, has only a one in three chance of being able to read and write when she grows up

The previous chapter sought to learn lessons from success, but for every Sri Lanka there are other poor countries where millions of people cannot afford to see a doctor, where their daughters have never been to school, and where their homes have neither taps nor toilets. Countries such as Yemen. A woman in Yemen has only a one in three chance of being able to read and write.[63] If she has a baby, she has only a one in five chance of being attended by a midwife.[64] If she and her child survive childbirth, the child has a one in three chance of being malnourished and a one in nine chance of dying before their fifth birthday.[65] If she lives in a rural area, her family is unlikely to be able to access medical care, clean water, or basic sanitation.[66]

Governments in poor countries have a clear responsibility to their citizens to provide health care, education, and water and sanitation to their people. They should do this not just because they have a duty and a responsibility to fulfil the human rights of their citizens, but also because it is in the long-term interests of the country and the economy to do so. Many governments in poor countries are simply failing to do this. The reality for the vast majority of poor people in developing countries is that they find public services either unavailable or dauntingly expensive and chronically under-staffed. What government spending there is goes disproportionately towards providing services such as hospitals and universities that mainly benefit the middle classes.

Lack of money is part of the reason for such failures, but lack of commitment is also to blame. Post-independence gains made from investing in essential services unravelled under the widespread economic crises of the 1970s and 1980s. The momentum for improving public services was

opposite page
Digging for water in Chulucanas, Peru. *'The water is OK for washing with, but it's not safe to drink'* — Juana Yorleque

lost by many governments, in some cases never to return, and the social contract unravelled as citizens came to expect little, and get less, from their governments. This chapter looks first at the impact of this neglect, and then at its causes.

Public sector heroes

'The shortages of nurses are really bad. You have to keep going even though you are very tired. I work from 4pm until 7.30am the next morning. That's 16 hours. There are five of us on the paediatric ward, and usually we have 200–300 kids. And I do day shifts covering for when we don't have enough people. We are hard-working; we are sweating. We keep going — what else can we do?'

Midwife in Lilongwe hospital, Malawi[67]

In many countries, where there is a lack of government cash or commitment, public services are kept afloat by a skeleton staff of overworked and underpaid teachers, doctors, nurses, administrators, engineers, and other public workers. Under appalling conditions, many workers do not do their jobs well or simply do not turn up. However, many more are committed to their work, putting in long hours with few resources and for little pay. For health workers these conditions can even be life-threatening — many risk HIV infection for want of disposable gloves, for instance. Given the circumstances, their commitment is nothing short of heroic.

Starvation wages

Teachers in the least developed countries once earned a good living, but their salaries have halved since 1970 (see Figure 4). This means that teachers and other public workers often do not get paid enough to survive on.

'I can tell you that I pay 300 cordobas ($18) for electricity, 250 ($14.50) for water, 300 for telephone; that's already half my salary and the rest of it goes on rice and beans, so there's nothing left for a bit of meat or anything else.'

Head teacher, José Madriz School, Nicaragua

Within the public sector, it is women who are in the lowest-paid and least-rewarded jobs. Sometimes these can literally be starvation wages. In Zambia, the Jesuit College for Theological Reflection calculated in May 2006 that the monthly cost of absolute basic needs for a family of six to survive was 1.4 million kwacha ($410). An average teacher's salary was 660,000 kwacha ($191) and an average nurse's salary was 1.2 million kwacha ($351).[68]

Low wages, weak management, and corruption discourages people from entering public services. In 2001 the government of Kenya advertised 100 doctor vacancies, but only eight people applied.[69]

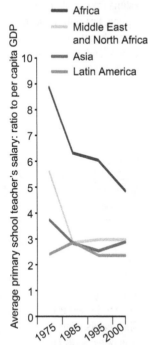

Figure 4: Falling salaries

— Africa
— Middle East and North Africa
— Asia
— Latin America

Average primary school teacher's salary: ratio to per capita GDP

(Source: UNESCO, Education For All Global Monitoring Report 2005)

Box 1: Public sector heroes

Around the world teachers, doctors, and nurses work long hours in terrible conditions and are paid a pittance. These are the unsung heroes working to do their best in crumbling public services.

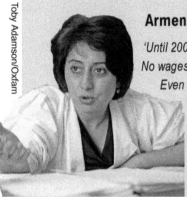

Armenia

'Until 2000, there was nothing. No wages, no drugs, and no facilities. Even since then, we have debts to pay for wages. Still I lack the equipment and diagnostics; I get the training but then I don't have the tools. But I am trained as a doctor; I should work. It is my moral duty. If people are ill I have to help somehow, even without the drugs being available. There are a lot of heroes here but their salaries don't match what the doctors do.'

Aregar Baghdasaryan, a doctor at Vayk polyclinic

Bangladesh

'I serve 100–150 patients a week and they come to get treatment for TB, family planning, or diarrhoea. I come from this area and know the people here. I spend the average day worrying because of financial hardship. I do not take fees from the patients. The primary reason for being a health worker is to serve the people.'

Beauty Mandal, health worker

Nicaragua

'I know people who are now qualified, and that makes me happy: seeing what I brought about. They say to me, "Teacher, if you hadn't behaved in such and such a way,I wouldn't have learned anything". And I appreciate that. It's my mission and vocation. I like teaching and that keeps me going. I'm now 60 and every year, when I get desperate because no-one wants to help me and I feel I'm drowning, I say I'm going to retire.'

Martha Ruiz, head teacher from a primary school at León, Nicaragua

Liberia

'The school is in need of so many things. There are no textbooks, no chairs or benches — you can see for yourself. But I am satisfied with the job I am doing. I am not teaching because of the pay but because I love the job and I love children. As long as there is breath in my body, I will continue to teach.'

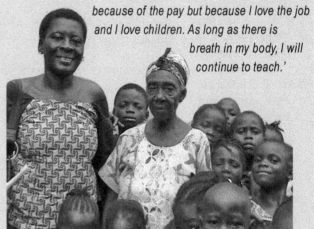

Mother Viola Shaw-Lewis, 76-year-old teacher at Kingsville public school, Liberia

Kenya

'I became a doctor because I want to help my people. I am a Turkana and I grew up experiencing the same problems. I therefore want to make a difference through my work as a doctor. Because of the harsh climatic conditions in Turkana, many professionals do not like working here, and this limits services to the people. I do not mind working here because I grew up in the same environment and, first and foremost, I have a call to serve my people.'

Dr. Yakish Eyapan, Lodwar District Hospital

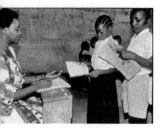

Mrs. Mwabuga is a
teacher at Uhuru primary
school, Shinyanga town,
Tanzania.
*'When I started in the
1970s, I was teaching a
class of 45 pupils.
Now it can be 180 or 200.
It's like a public meeting:
we give a speech, it's
not teaching'*

The missing millions — doctors, nurses, teachers, and administrators

The past 30 years have bequeathed a legacy of neglect. Today many governments lack the money and the workforce to build public services up to the scale and quality required.

Globally there are shortages of 4.25 million health workers[70] and 1.9 million teachers[71] — the biggest single obstacle to scaling up essential services and to tackling HIV/AIDS.[72]

Some countries are suffering more than others. In Nepal, there are on average 180 children per trained teacher (see Figure 5). Oxfam has calculated that:

Teachers

Based on the Education For All target of a minimum of one trained teacher for every 40 school-age children:[73]

- At least 30 countries in the world do not have enough trained primary school teachers to educate their children.

- In 11 of these countries, there are not enough teachers for more than half of the school-age children.

Figure 5: Missing teachers

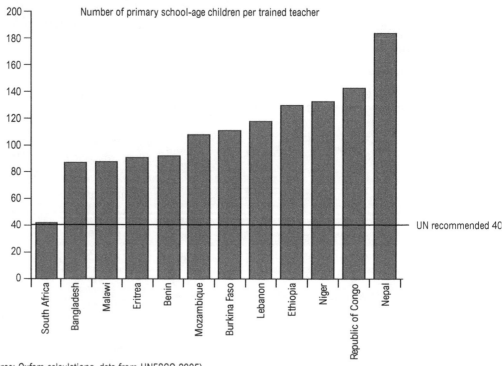

(Source: Oxfam calculations, data from UNESCO 2005)

Figure 6: Missing health workers

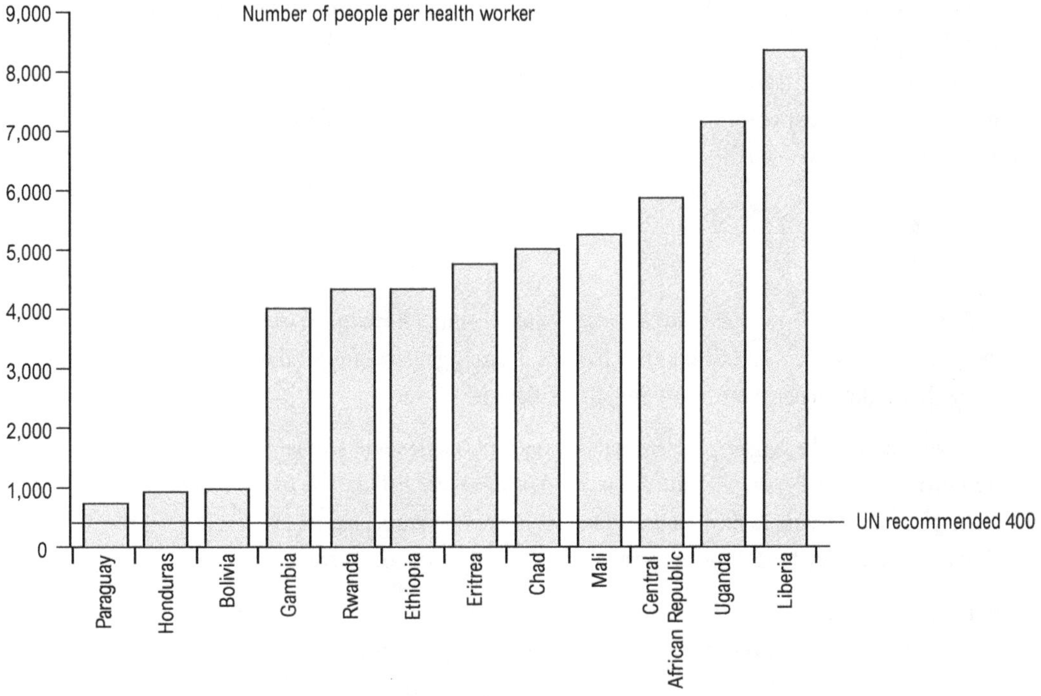

Number of people per health worker

(Source: Oxfam calculations, based on data from Joint Learning Initiative 2004)

Health workers

Based on a minimum standard of 2.5 health workers per 1,000 population:[74]

- At least 75 countries do not have enough trained health workers to meet their needs.
- Of these, 53 countries have fewer than half the trained health workers needed.
- In 10 countries,[75] there are only enough trained health workers to cover 10 per cent of the population (see Figure 6).

HIV/AIDS redoubles the challenge. Africa is likely to lose 20 per cent of its health workers to the disease over the coming few years, with those remaining facing increased workloads and stress.[76] In Malawi, 25–30 per cent of health professionals will die of AIDS in the next decade — 'and before they die, they are sick and can't work'.[77] With painful irony, this undermines the country's efforts to expand the provision of ARV treatment to people living with HIV and AIDS. 'As much as we want to scale up, there are no bodies,' said Biswick Mwale, head of Malawi's National AIDS Commission. 'People can't translate money into action when there are no people.'[78]

'As much as we want to scale up, there are no bodies,' said Biswick Mwale, head of Malawi's National AIDS Commission. 'People can't translate money into action when there are no people.'

Leaving for a better life

Many public workers have left to work in the local private sector, or to work overseas. Around 50 per cent of Africa's medical graduates go overseas within five years of finishing their studies.[79] Most head for Europe and the USA, which are home to 20 per cent of the world's people, almost 50 per cent of the world's physicians, and 60 per cent of its nurses.[80] This issue is discussed further in section 4.

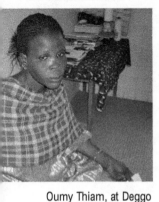

Oumy Thiam, at Deggo
Health Centre, Dakar,
Senegal.
*'I am four months pregnant
and until now I have
consulted neither a
physician nor a midwife
because I cannot afford it.
Fortunately [the nurse] has
agreed to treat me.
For me, the government is
responsible for ensuring
that we have access to
health services.
So, if the authorities are
really committed, they
should provide people like
me with free health care'*

Killer fees

'My husband and I are unemployed, we have no income. I have to beg the nursing officer to treat me free of charge because I cannot pay the fees. I rarely go to the hospital because of lack of means.'
Oumy Thiam (four months pregnant) from Dakar, Senegal

'For the children the biggest problem is that they have no books or clothes. Despite the government's commitment to universal free education, poor children are still unable to come to school. They go around trying to find money so they can buy books and return to school.'
Justin Zimba, deputy head of Makangwse Open Community School, Zambia

Where states lack the capacity or commitment to fund services, poor people are made to pay instead. User fees are a life-or-death issue for people from Ethiopia to Georgia (see Box 2), and making households pay excludes women and girls, who are usually last in line for services.[81] Although fees rarely contribute more than 5 per cent[82] of running costs for health and education systems, they have proliferated in all regions. Despite widely recognised gains in countries that have abolished fees in primary education, 89 out of 103 countries surveyed by the World Bank for UNESCO still levy official or informal charges for schooling.[83] Botswana and South Africa have recently made disappointing U-turns by reintroducing tuition fees in education; many other countries charge for uniforms and textbooks, which are a similar burden for poor people. In the poorest countries, total out-of-pocket health spending can be two to three times greater than government spending on health.[84]

In water services, unlike in health and education, user fees are needed in order to encourage sustainable use of finite water resources. It is crucial, however, that tariffs are structured to ensure that a minimum daily amount of water is free or affordable for poor people.

Box 2: Pay, or stay away

User fees do not work: they exclude poor people from the services they need most.

Women bear the greatest burden of user fees. Their reproductive role means that they have the greatest need of public services, but in many societies their low status and lack of income mean they are last in line for medical care and schooling. This is exacerbated where people have to pay for services. Studies suggest that user fees result in higher maternal and infant mortality rates — in one Nigerian district, the numbers of women dying in childbirth doubled after fees were introduced for maternal health services, and the number of babies delivered in hospitals declined by half.[85] Similar results have been observed in Tanzania and Zimbabwe.[86]

Eighteen-year-old Clémentine, from Cibitoke in Burundi, recounted the impact user fees had on her and her newborn baby: '*After the delivery I was presented with a bill for 30,900F [around $30]. As I didn't have anything to pay with, I was imprisoned in the health centre... I remained there for a week, in detention, without care and without food. I was suffering from anaemia and my baby had respiratory and digestive problems.*'[87]

Burundi introduced fees to cover the full cost of consultations and medicines in 2002 — supported by the World Bank and the IMF. Two years later, a survey found that less than 1 per cent of patients were exempt, and that average fees exceeded two weeks' wages for agricultural workers. As a result, four out of five patients had gone into debt or had sold some of their harvest to raise the money needed for their treatment. When patients did not pay, clinics imprisoned them or seized their identity papers. It was little surprise that the number of women dying in childbirth rose after the charges were introduced.[88]

Révérien explained the consequences for his family: '*My wife died a few months ago. Very probably from malaria because she had a lot of fever and was also vomiting. But I don't know, since she never went to the health centre as we didn't have enough money. I don't even have enough to feed my two children, so how could I have paid the price of a consultation? I thought that she would eventually get better. That didn't happen. After four months in that state, she died.*'[89]

In February 2006 the Burundian government abolished charges for maternity and child care services, but it has still to extend free care to other basic health-care services.

In Georgia, the introduction of fees for all but the most basic health treatments has stopped many people from seeking medical help. '*I have only a small pension, no other income, so it's almost impossible,*' said Gvinianidze Taili, a 75-year-old woman from Tbilisi. '*I would definitely use the clinic more often if it was free.*' Hospital admission rates fell by two-thirds between 1990 and 1999 and outpatient services fell by four-fifths, following a dramatic drop in health service funding.[90] The number of people using the health service fell from a level that was equivalent to use in Western Europe to a level closer to that of sub-Saharan Africa.

Fees are also distorting medical practice. '*We have two patients at the moment who need urgent operations and they can't get them,*' said Nana Ckhadadic, a therapist in a Tbilisi clinic. '*It's a hard situation to be in for a doctor. You have to diagnose not just their illness but their ability to pay, and then try and fit this to the free treatments that are available from the state programmes. Anything vaguely similar to cardiovascular disease gets diagnosed as cardiovascular disease, because that's an illness covered by the state programme. That's why everything should be free.*'[91]

Fees can also undermine the benefits of progress in other areas. A World Bank study of recent successes in reducing maternal mortality in Bolivia, China, Egypt, Honduras, Indonesia, and Zimbabwe found that the presence of trained birth attendants at community health centres was central to such success. But it also concluded that these countries are unlikely to reduce maternal mortality as quickly as Sri Lanka or Malaysia because they charge fees, which are a '*substantial and a major deterrent to use*'.[92]

Sources: Médecins Sans Frontières 2004 and Belli, P., Shahriari, H. and Curtio Medical Group 2002

Non-state providers are picking up some of the pieces

Non-state providers (NSPs) fill some of the gaps when states fail to provide essential services. NSPs range from civil society organisations such as non-government organisations (NGOs), churches, mosques, and community organisations to profit-making companies, and in size from individual street traders to multinational corporations. Some aim to supply schooling and clinics for the wealthy end of the market; others focus on meeting the needs of low-income families.

In Nigeria, faith-based organisations provide 60 per cent of health care; in Malawi NGOs provide over 30 per cent.

The services provided by NSPs — both private providers and non-profit organisations — are crucial for millions of people. Across ten cities in Africa, for example, the main water sources for an average 47 per cent of households are small-scale providers or traditional wells.[93] In South-East Asian cities, small-scale water providers serve 20–45 per cent of households.[94] In Nigeria, faith-based organisations (FBOs) provide 60 per cent of health care; in Malawi NGOs provide over 30 per cent.[95]

Primary education typically is publicly provided, but community and NGO-run schools are important in several countries. Two-thirds of primary schools in Malawi are owned by the church and in Bangladesh about one schoolchild in four attends a non-government primary school (some 60 per cent of these are run by a single organisation, the Bangladesh Rural Advancement Committee, or BRAC).[96]

Non-profit providers have distinct advantages. Some pilot and promote innovative practices which can be adopted by the state, for example in the area of gender-based violence, where close co-ordination between the health, police, and judicial authorities is crucial. Many are good at reaching remote and marginalised communities or at providing community-based services, such as home-based care for AIDS sufferers. Moreover, many civil society organisations support citizens to claim their rights on health and education — for example, through community radio programmes and support for the empowerment of girls and the development of leadership among women.

In the absence of public services, many communities build their own schools, dig their own wells, and care for their sick as best as they can. Some in-kind contributions from communities can be helpful — such as labour and materials for school construction or for maintaining community water points. But making up for weak public services puts a heavy burden on communities, and most simply do not have the resources to provide decent quality services — as Jennifer Chiwela, chairperson of the Zambian National Education Coalition, explained:

> *'Since the mid-1990s, the government has been unable to meet its responsibility to educate our children. Communities rose to that need and began to bring their children together to get some form of education. These schools take many forms, and conditions vary greatly. Some are good schools, but others, many of them, really leave much to be desired. They don't have sufficient learning materials, books, pencils, pens. They may not even have proper sanitation.'*

Elsewhere, the heavy presence of for-profit providers results in inequalities in access and in the quality of services, based on the ability to pay. Poor people in the cities of Accra and Dar es Salaam pay up to five times more for a litre of water than other users because they have to buy it from private vendors who are not regulated by the government in their pricing or service quality.[97]

Typically, government regulation of the many different types of NSP exists primarily on paper, and often focuses on regulating entry into the sector and monitoring the inputs used, rather than on the quality of services provided.[98] When there is no clear government policy framework for working with NSPs, the result is a patchwork of provision — a lottery for citizens, depending on where they live and what they can afford.

When there is no clear government policy framework for working with NSPs, the result is a patchwork of provision.

The key causes of this terrible situation are outlined below — but, in brief, they are not enough money, money poorly spent, and systems that are often undermined by corruption.

Missing money

Although a great deal can be achieved at low cost if money is spent well, there is no doubt that this crisis has been caused partly by a chronic lack of funding in developing countries. Spending on essential services has been growing in recent years, but for most countries it is nowhere near fast enough to meet the MDGs. The need for services continues to grow, with rising populations and the impact of HIV/AIDS — but in many countries economic growth is low and governments simply cannot keep up.

Basic education, of all the basic services, has received financial priority over the past decade, with spending rising most years in most countries.[99] Around half of African countries are now spending a higher percentage of their budget on education than high-income countries in North America and Europe are.[100] However, globally, up to $17 billion extra per year is still needed to put every child in a decent primary school — of which at least $10 billion will need to come from rich countries by 2010.[101]

Globally, up to $17 billion extra per year is still needed to put every child in a decent primary school.

Health spending in poor countries has also increased in the past ten years, thanks to new funds for HIV/AIDS, but new money is needed to tackle basic health problems such as measles and diarrhoea, which also kill many children. Government health spending in low-income countries has increased over the past decade from a low base,[102] but most countries will require substantial external assistance to reach even the recommended minimum of $34 per person per year (see Figure 7).[103]

Figure 7: Minimum health spending: some regions are a long way off

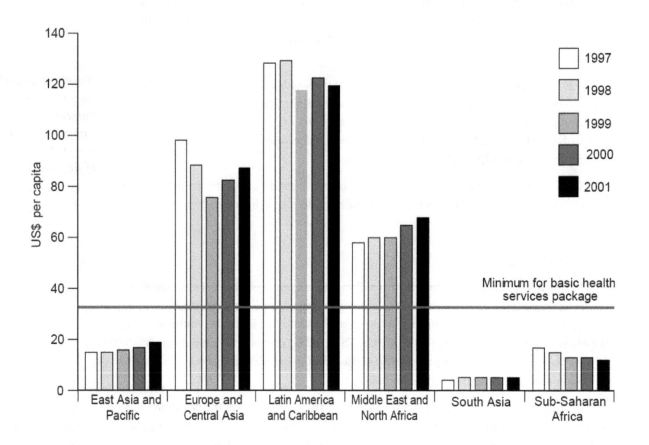

(Source: WHO 2004 in Global Monitoring Report 2005)

Current investments in water and sanitation in developing countries amount to $14–16 billion per year. At least double that amount is needed to reach the MDGs, and much more if broader sanitation and sustainable water management targets are included.[104] Overall, as Figure 8 shows, many countries will need to double what governments and rich country aid donors currently spend in order to attain the MDGs. Governments in the poorest countries simply cannot afford to do this alone — just providing a minimum health-care package would use up most of their current tax revenues.[105]

Figure 8: Falling far short: missing money for the MDGs

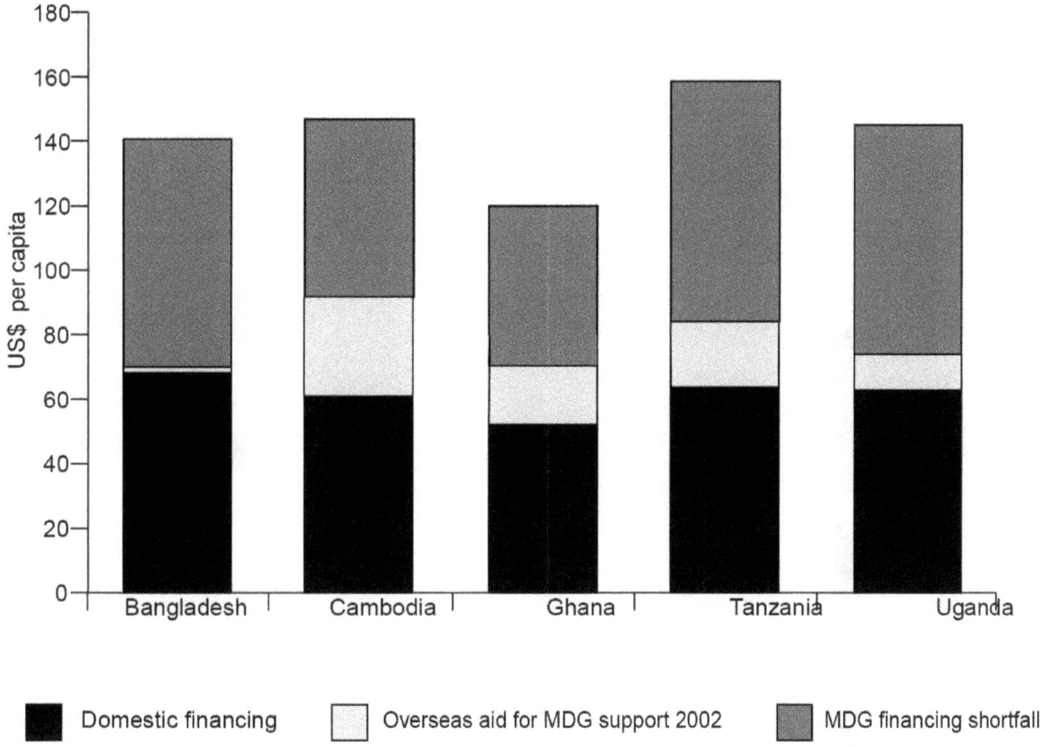

(Source: UN Millennium Project 2005b)

Some governments could do more with the money they have. In Abuja, Nigeria in 2001, African countries committed themselves to spending a larger share on health — at least 15 per cent of their budgets. However, to date only Mozambique and the Democratic Republic of Congo have met this commitment. Health spending has actually declined in seven of these African countries (Seychelles, Namibia, Lesotho, South Africa, Zimbabwe, Madagascar, and Botswana).

And while security is a legitimate concern, some governments are putting excessive spending on the latest military hardware before people's lives. Thirty-six countries in the world spend more on their military forces than they do on health or education. Figure 9 shows the size of military spending in the ten countries with the weakest human development records.[106]

Figure 9: Guns not schools — the ten worst offenders

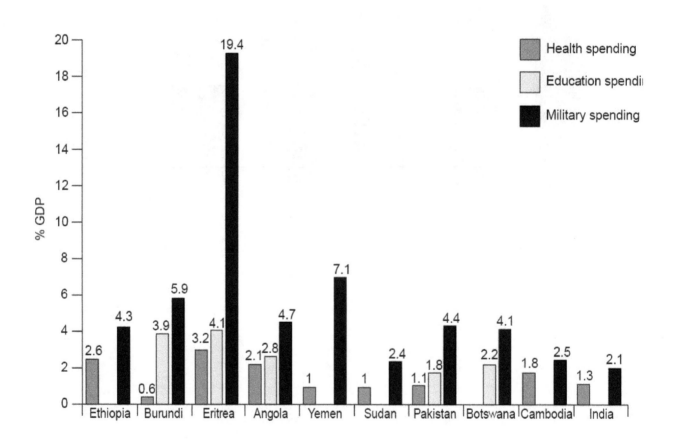

(Source: Oxfam calculations, based on data from UNDP 2005)

The problem of the lack of money for essential services is compounded by inefficiencies and inequalities in the way it is used.

Servicing the rich

Successful countries concentrate their public spending on primary services and in rural areas, where most of the world's poor people live. Unfortunately in many countries a larger proportion of money is spent on services used by a wealthy minority, such as prestigious universities, city hospitals, or piped water supplies that never reach poor neighbourhoods or rural areas.[107] In a World Bank study of 35 developing countries, only a handful of countries succeeded in directing as much or more public health and education spending to the poorest fifth of society as to the richest fifth.[108]

Many countries in Latin America slip under the MDG radar because their aggregate development data compare well with other regions. However, this masks deeply engrained inequalities within countries. The education gap between rural and urban children in Nicaragua and Honduras is greater than for children in far poorer countries such as Kenya, Viet Nam, and Guyana.[109] In Ecuador, the poorest 25 per cent of six-year-olds score so far behind their richer peers in simple vocabulary recognition tests, that '*it is uncertain whether and how they could ever catch up*'.[110] Indigenous populations in rural areas are too often ignored when it comes to public services. Half of household heads in rural Guatemala have no education, compared with one-fifth in urban areas.[111]

In Nepal, more than 60 per cent of investments in water supply and sanitation will go to provide services to just 6 per cent of the country's population. This is largely because of an expensive water pipeline project in the capital Kathmandu, which is costing $312 per capita, while only $16 per person is spent in rural areas.[112]

In countries such as Peru, Guatemala, Mali, Morocco, and the Philippines, women from the richest fifth of households are around seven times more likely than women from the poorest fifth to be assisted by a skilled health worker when giving birth — and so are far less likely to die or to lose their baby (see Figure 10).

In Nepal, more than 60 per cent of investment in water supply and sanitation will go to provide services to just 6 per cent of the country's population.

Figure 10: Giving birth, rich and poor

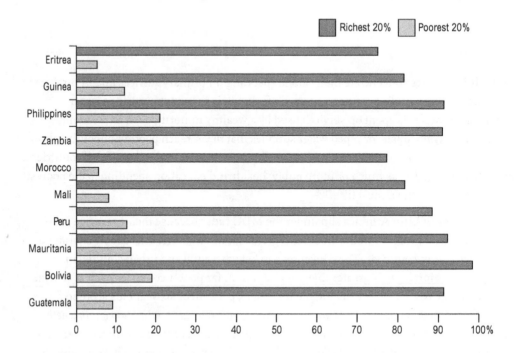

Percentage of births attended by skilled health personnel, by richest and poorest fifths of society

(Source: data from Human Development Report 2005)

This problem is chronic in India — home to one-third of the world's poor people — where millions lack access to essential services. China and India are in the front rank of high-growth, globalising countries. Yet progress in reducing child deaths has slowed in both countries to such an extent that lower-income Viet Nam and Bangladesh have overtaken their larger neighbours in improving child mortality rates.[113]

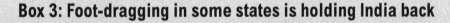

Box 3: Foot-dragging in some states is holding India back

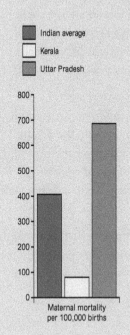

- Indian average
- Kerala
- Uttar Pradesh

Maternal mortality
per 100,000 births

Despite recent economic growth and government promises to increase health and education spending and to cut infant deaths, India remains a country of deep inequalities, entrenched by its previous failure to invest comprehensively in rural development.

India produces some of the most highly qualified doctors and engineers, yet it has the largest number of people unable to read or write. Girls born in Uttar Pradesh state are five times more likely to die before their fifth birthday, half as likely to become literate, and likely to live 20 years less than girls born in Kerala — where the state government has made essential services a priority.[114] The Indian government continues to spend almost twice as much on its military forces as it does on health.[115]

Figure 11:
Surviving childbirth depends on where you live

(Source: Indian National Health Policy, 2002)

The curse of corruption

> *'Corruption is commonplace. A lot of abuses are going on with the stealing of drugs, and equipment being taken from our health centres and put into private clinics. We don't have the human resources needed to put the necessary checks and balances in place. Our systems are terribly, terribly weak.'*
> Technical adviser, ministry of health, African government[116]

Corruption is a major problem in the provision of essential services. This is true in rich and poor countries alike. In the USA, the Attorney General has declared health-care fraud to be the country's 'number two crime problem' after violent crime, costing billions each year. In Cambodia, private companies frequently pay substantial bribes to obtain government contracts.[117] Across the developing world, informal 'fees' are charged for water, education, and health services.[118]

Corruption has the biggest impact on the poorest people, who are the first to suffer from the denial of services. In Romania, a World Bank study showed that the poorest third of families pay 11 per cent of their income in bribes, while the richest third pay just 2 per cent.[119]

Corruption can be a problem in essential services regardless of whether the services are privately or publicly provided,[120] but the kind of corruption differs depending on the system. Where providers are private but are funded publicly, corruption is mainly about overcharging governments and failing to deliver quality services. This is particularly likely where government capacity for oversight and the enforcement of contracts is weak. In Nicaragua, for instance, over $600,000 was lost following poorly regulated contracts with private sector contractors to build and maintain schools.[121]

In situations where the public sector is the provider, corruption takes different forms, such as illegal fees and bribes for services; absenteeism and staff taking second jobs in the private sector; funds going missing while being transferred from central to local government; bribes being paid to secure positions or promotion; and the creation of 'ghost workers' to divert payrolls. In Honduras a World Bank study found that 7.6 per cent of public sector staff either did not exist or had moved to other posts.[122]

In the worst instances a vicious circle is created, where a culture of impunity further weakens already crumbling public systems through bribery and misappropriation. A population starved of information and of any opportunity to have its complaints heard or acted upon eventually becomes resigned to poor or non-existent services.

Conclusion

Governments have a duty to provide health care, education, and water and sanitation to their people. But too many governments are failing to deliver on that duty — because they lack the cash, the capacity, or the commitment. Faced with this failure, many poor people are reliant on non-profit or private providers of variable quality, or are themselves struggling to provide services as best they can. Governments need to build strong public systems that can provide good quality services to their citizens. In many countries fulfilling this duty means working with non-state providers to integrate and regulate them properly within public systems. In all of this, the role of development partners is crucial — but how good are rich country governments at supporting public services?

4

Rich country governments:

pushing for private provision, and breaking aid promises

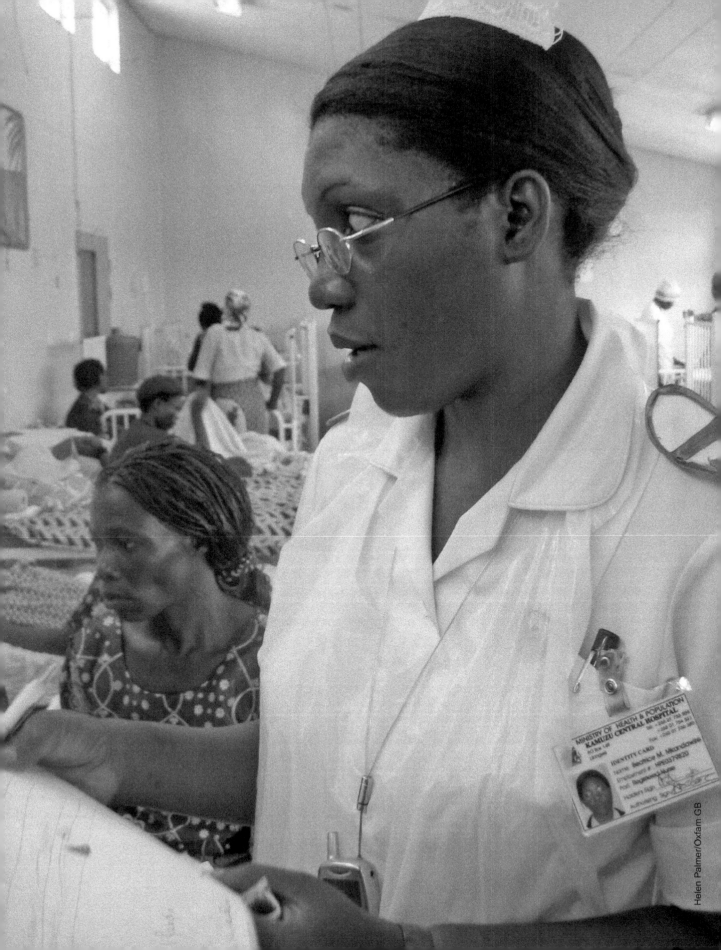

4
Rich country governments: pushing for private provision, and breaking aid promises

While poor country governments can make or break progress in delivering decent health care, education, and water and sanitation to their people, rich country governments also have a great, and often decisive, influence. For some of the poorest countries, donor aid is equivalent to half the government budget. In others, donor-funded technical assistance can drive a reform agenda. But instead of using their influence to revitalise public services, rich country governments too often push private sector solutions to public service failures, despite the evidence that this does not work. Many rich countries are also guilty of poaching health workers and teachers from poor countries. And they are giving too little aid, too late, and in the wrong ways. This chapter briefly reviews the evidence on private provision, and explores the role of rich country governments, the World Bank, and the IMF.

Private provision is profitable, but not equitable

Some countries have achieved impressive welfare gains with a high level of private involvement in service delivery. South Korea and Chile both have private health insurance systems, with the government funding health care for the poorest people, while Chile's private water utility provides safe water to 97 per cent of its urban population and sanitation to 90 per cent.[123] In neither case has the state abdicated overall responsibility — strong public regulation has been key to their success. However, even in countries such as these, with an effective civil service, essential services are prone to high inequalities, high costs, and skewed provision, because private providers are notoriously hard to regulate.

Inequalities in access to health care in Chile grew during the 1980s, when public funding was reduced during the country's economic crisis.[124] Chile has the highest rate of births by Caesarean section in the world (40 per cent in 1997) because private hospitals benefit from the extra costs of surgery and higher bed occupancy rates.[125] Private service provision can go badly wrong when profit motives make services unaffordable for poor people, when companies dictate contractual terms, and when governments lack the capacity to regulate effectively.

opposite page
Another busy day for Nurse Beatrice Mkandawire at Kamuzu Central Hospital, Malawi.
'The nurse/patient ratio we have, it's too big. Medicines are also a big problem. It's very hard. But I'm not leaving. If all of us go, who's going to look after all of these mothers and small children?'

Excluding poor people

Privately-provided services are usually too expensive for poor people. In the 1990s in China, where hospitals are run on a for-profit basis, up to 40 per cent of people in rural areas did not seek health care because they could not afford it — a situation that still affects millions today (see Box 4).[126]

Lucrative contracts for corporations

When multinational companies enter into contracts with low-income and low-capacity governments, the imbalance of power can easily lead to abuse. The water market worldwide is dominated by a handful of US, French, and UK companies, such as Bechtel, Suez, and Biwater. When these companies negotiate contracts in developing countries they often 'cherry pick' the most profitable market segments and require guaranteed profit margins, denominated in dollars.[127] The firms can also insist on full cost recovery, which inevitably hikes up prices for poor people.

If governments try to terminate these contracts, they risk being sued. In the late 1990s, the World Bank and the IMF demanded water privatisation in Cochabamba, Bolivia, as a condition for debt relief and new loans.[128] AdT, the consortium involved — partly owned by US-based Bechtel and Edison of Italy[129] —was guaranteed profits in its 40-year contract with the government.[130] Under AdT's management the price of water increased drastically,[131] to the point that it cost the average family living on the local minimum wage up to 25 per cent of its monthly income.[132] Such unaffordable prices triggered huge public protests.[133] The Bolivian government subsequently terminated the contract, and the companies involved attempted to sue the government for $25 million.[134] After huge public pressure and negative publicity, Bechtel dropped the case.[135]

Box 4: Uninsured and untreated in China

Jin Guilian lies in an unheated and poorly equipped clinic, suffering from congenital heart disease and a blackened, festering arm. His only treatment is oxygen and a saline drip. He is a migrant labourer, and his employer evaded paying his health insurance, so now his family have to pay for treatment themselves. His relatives took him back home, 500 miles by bus, to the cheapest clinic they could find. '*If he dies, he'll die here. If he recovers, he'll recover here,*' said his brother. '*We don't have any other means.*'

China's health sector reforms have required hospitals to operate for profit, charging market prices for drugs and operations. Services that were once free are now paid for through health insurance — but 80 per cent of the rural population, like Jin Guilian, are not insured. The result? Household costs for health care rose forty-fold between 1989 and 2002. The devastating impacts are clear for individuals like Jin Guilian.

Source: French, H. '*Wealth grows, but health care withers in China*', *New York Times*, 14 January 2006

Water privatisation is the most notorious example, but private sector involvement in health care is also spreading rapidly, in many cases with little regulation. Experience in some of the first countries to implement reforms of this nature echoes that of the water sector. Chile was one of the first countries to implement private sector involvement in its health-care system. It soon became clear that the private sector was 'skimming the risk pool' by catering to the needs of the young and healthy, while providing services to just 2 per cent of people aged over 65. The interests of the private sector were clearly demonstrated when one private insurer closed its plans to women aged 18–45, following the withdrawal of the government maternity subsidy.[136] A health law was passed in 2002 seeking to redress this injustice, by giving more powers to government to regulate the private sector and to build public sector capacity.

Despite it being one of the foremost proponents of private sector solutions, the World Bank's own research has revealed the weakness of crude 'private good, public bad' approaches. A 2002 World Bank study of Asian and Pacific water companies found that *'efficiency is not significantly different in private companies than in public ones'*.[137] A more recent Bank survey of econometric studies likewise concluded that ownership does not matter as much as is sometimes argued: *'Most cross-country papers on utilities find no statistical difference in efficiency scores between public and private providers.'*[138] What does matter is the cost of the service for poor people, but another Bank-funded study of private utility provision found that *'efficiency gains were achieved at the cost of an increase in the burden imposed on the lowest income groups connected'*.[139] In other words, poor people pay more.

As the example of Chile shows, the key to making private provision work lies in the state's ability to regulate, but this is often exactly what is lacking. And there is a high price attached to its absence: weak monitoring capacity in the government of Guinea, for example, led to a private water contractor receiving double the compensation originally expected.[140] The irony is that where state services are weakest, so is the state's capacity to regulate others — which is why simply giving up on the state and betting on the private sector does not work.

The key to making private provision work lies in the state's ability to regulate, but this is often exactly what is lacking.

Pushing for private

The predilection of aid providers for market solutions is a direct echo of debates going on in many rich countries themselves. At first the debate focused primarily on wholesale privatisation, but recently this has moved into the more nuanced terrain of public–private partnerships (PPPs). These involve elements of service provision being contracted out to private sector providers or to charities, churches, and NGOs; or they involve other ways of introducing market-like behaviour into public services, for example through increased autonomy and competition between individual hospitals or schools. This approach to services is known as New Public Management (NPM) and was first introduced in New Zealand, where it had alarming impacts in terms of costs, waiting times, and poor people's access to services.[141] One of NPM's key proponents, Allen Shick, has urged developing countries not to attempt reforms of this nature.[142]

Given the abundant historical evidence of governments stepping in to provide services precisely because of failures in the market (see chapter 2), the burden of proof for this return to market and private sector solutions should lie squarely with those who advocate it. Instead, the opposite has been the case. The market and private providers are consistently assumed to be more efficient and effective, while the public sector is presumed guilty of incurable inefficiency and ineptitude.

In fact the evidence is much more mixed. Studies of efficiency show that while the public sector is indeed failing in many countries, unconditional surrender to market forces does little to guarantee success. A recent IMF paper looked at public–private partnerships in utilities and concluded: '*Much of the case for PPPs rests on the relative efficiency of the private sector. While there is extensive literature on the subject, the theory is ambiguous and the evidence is mixed.*'[143] A recent review of private sector participation in education and health reached similar conclusions.[144] Private sector or market-based reforms have delivered services more effectively only where there have been strong and enforceable regulations, competitive markets, and well-informed consumers — all of which are noticeably absent in most developing countries.

Despite the evidence that it is government action and not the market that has been behind the universal provision of essential services in successful countries, the World Bank and its sister organisation, the International Monetary Fund (IMF), together with many bilateral aid donors, appear determined to push increased private provision of services as their default policy position.

Loans with strings

Privatisation is still a condition in multilateral lending to the poorest countries.

A 2006 survey of countries receiving IMF and World Bank loans found that 18 out of 20 faced conditions requiring privatisation.

- A 2005 study of the World Bank's latest adjustment loans, the Poverty Reduction Support Credits, found that 11 out of 13 schemes studied contained conditions. These included water privatisation in Nicaragua and greater involvement of the private sector in health-care provision in Senegal.[147]

- A 2006 survey of countries receiving IMF and World Bank loans found that 18 out of 20 faced conditions requiring privatisation, an increase on previous years.[148]

- A 2006 study of debt cancellation found that reforms requiring some form of privatisation were a pre-condition for debt relief in over half the countries that qualified for the Highly Indebted Poor Countries (HIPC)[149] initiative.[150]

Ganging up

The World Bank promotes the private provision of basic services through interlocking conditions on aid and debt relief to poor countries.[151] This appears to be driven more by the Bank's internal targets than by evidence of what works in each country — for example, the Bank's Private Sector Development Strategy aims for private sector participation in 40 per cent

Box 5: The World Bank and the private sector[145]

The World Bank is the most influential voice in international aid policy, and its annual flagship, the World Development Report (WDR), is its most important publication. The strong bias within the Bank towards market and private sector solutions to public service reform is evident from its 2004 World Development Report, *Making Services Work for Poor People*.

The report's premise is that the widespread failure of basic services to work for poor people is primarily a crisis of accountability, which is best resolved by a smaller role for the state and the marketisation of service delivery. This is epitomised in the WDR's 'eight sizes fit all' model,[146] which experiments with varying degrees of contracting out services to private and non-profit providers.

The problem with this approach is that it both fails to identify other, equally important causes of service failure and is heavily biased towards market-based reforms that are unproven and inappropriate in many countries, even for improving accountability.

It is true that lack of accountability is a major barrier to improving the access, quality, equity, and efficiency of public services for poor people. But lack of cash and the capacity to deliver services are equally important. As well as better mechanisms for accountability and participation in

service delivery, public services also need top-level political commitment from government; progressive and stable taxation systems; decent levels of spending; well-motivated and well-paid public sector workers and managers; and citizens who expect and demand well-performing public services as a right. To any of these problems, contracting out service delivery, voucher schemes, and various other market-based 'accountability' measures are poor and in some cases counter-productive solutions.

Ultimately the role of the World Bank and other development institutions should lie in helping to strengthen effective public services, rather than trying to circumvent them by parcelling out government responsibilities to the private sector.

It is important to recognise that the World Bank is far from monolithic — its staff display a wide range of opinion on the private versus public debate and the Bank has clearly learned some lessons from the past failures of its structural adjustment programmes. The World Bank as an institution, though, shows little sign of abandoning its more rigid ideological stance, and there is often a serious gap between the relatively nuanced debate in its headquarters in Washington and its much more heavy-handed approach on the ground.

of its loans to the poorest countries.[152] The Bank's private sector lender, the International Finance Corporation (IFC), is forging ahead with private sector involvement in health care in 17 countries — including China, Côte d'Ivoire, and Colombia[153] — despite criticisms that previous IFC-backed investments have served only the wealthier end of the market.[154]

The IFC and the Bank's Multilateral Investment Guarantee Agency (MIGA), together with the export credit agencies of rich countries, are also encouraging private investors to get involved in services by promising firms compensation for losses if the poor country governments cancel contracts.[155] After the World Bank made privatisation of the Dar es Salaam Water And Sewerage Authority (DAWASA) in Tanzania a condition of HIPC debt relief, in November 2001 the UK's Export Credit Guarantee Department insured Biwater, a British company, for £2 million against risks of expropriation and restrictions on profits for its water utility operations in the country. By 2005 Biwater's project was well behind schedule and no new pipes had been installed,[156] but the company was suing the Tanzanian government for cancelling its contract.[157]

Ignoring public opinion

Insisting on privatisation also risks driving a wedge between governments and their people. Public opposition to privatisation is growing around the world. In a 2001 survey in 17 Latin American countries, privatisation was seen as 'not beneficial' by almost two-thirds of respondents.[158] A 2005 study identified 22 countries where citizens are actively opposing, or have halted, privatisation of water or energy.[159] Yet rich country governments are pressing on, aiming to change public opinion rather than their own approach. In 1999 the UK government paid Adam Smith International $1.3m to run publicity campaigns in Tanzania, extolling the virtues of privatisation.[160] The lyrics to its Tanzanian pop video claimed '*Our old industries are dry like crops and privatisation brings the rain.*'[161]

Trade agreements may threaten public services

Developing country governments are increasingly obliged to make policy within a web of constraints imposed by the World Trade Organisation, regional trade agreements, and bilateral investment treaties. These intrude well beyond border issues such as tariffs, into the spheres of domestic regulation and the provision of public services. In particular, such agreements limit how governments can regulate foreign service providers — for example, one reading of the WTO's General Agreement on Trade in Services (GATS) is that unless the government is the sole supplier of an essential service such as water or education (which is seldom the case in developing countries), it can be pressured to open the sector to foreign providers under GATS.

Although GATS also recognises the 'right to regulate' of developing countries, it is unclear whether this is sufficient for them to withstand pressure from other countries to open up the provision of water and health care. Water is the essential service most likely to come under pressure from GATS: through the WTO, the European Commission has asked 72 countries to liberalise their water distribution systems. Fifty WTO members have also made some kind of commitment on health services. Oxfam believes that GATS and other trade and investment treaties can potentially be used to place undue pressure on developing countries to open their services to foreign suppliers, when it may not be wise to do so. Oxfam also believes that GATS provision can be abused to undermine the power of the state to regulate service provision in favour of ensuring universal and good quality access.

Things the rich countries don't try at home

Rich country governments have responded to the gathering evidence on privatisations gone wrong, albeit more often in word than in deed. The UK, Norway, and the European Commission (EC) now publicly reject the inclusion of privatisation as a condition for aid.[162] However, all three continue to channel resources to World Bank projects that actively promote private sector solutions, or link their aid to conditions imposed by the World Bank and the IMF.

Some governments would never permit this at home. In Sweden, Denmark, and Norway, water is provided exclusively by effective public services. A law recently passed in the Netherlands has made the private provision of water illegal. Yet the Dutch government, together with those of Sweden and Norway, is a major contributor to the Public-Private Infrastructure Advisory Facility (PPIAF) and the Private Infrastructure Development Group (PIDG), multi-donor institutions which actively advocate for private sector management of water and sanitation services in developing countries.

Contracting out to civil society organisations: only a partial solution

In many cases, contracting out services to the not-for-profit civil society sector is being promoted as an alternative both to failed state provision and failed for-profit private company provision. There are many different types of civil society provider. Christian churches provide the majority of health services in many African countries, where they often pre-date government. In other cases charities or NGOs have stepped in. In some post-conflict states, contracting out has led to a speedy scale-up in the provision of services. In Afghanistan, international NGOs have been contracted to provide basic health services to over 50 per cent of the country in less than four years — although a review highlighted fears of high transaction costs, poor regulation, and insufficient transparency and monitoring in this kind of contracting arrangement.[163]

Christian churches provide the majority of health services in many African countries. In other cases charities or NGOs have stepped in.

Civil society providers can be more innovative and can improve equity by reaching some of the poor people missed by state services. Non-profit health-care providers in Nigeria and Malawi, for example, actively target poor people and work in rural areas,[164] while village-based schools run by BRAC in Bangladesh use interactive, participatory teaching methods in schools that are located close to local communities in rural areas not served by the government. BRAC also runs health programmes across the country.[165]

A recent review of contracting out health provision to civil society in poor countries and regions, including Cambodia, Bangladesh, Costa Rica, and South Africa,[166] concluded that some contracting out improved service delivery dramatically. However, since such contracts have often been introduced where public provision was virtually absent, no meaningful comparison could be made.[167] According to other studies, contracting out has been successful largely because staff have been paid higher wages, civil society providers have had additional

In Cambodia, the increase in service uptake by poor people was attributable largely to the reduction in out-of-pocket costs for patients and the higher wages paid to staff.

resources, or providers have abolished user fees. In Cambodia, the increase in service uptake by poor people achieved in contracted-out health clinics was attributable largely to the reduction in out-of-pocket costs for patients and the higher wages paid to staff — presumably an outcome also possible in government clinics, had government staff been paid market rates and fees been abolished.[168]

As with the for-profit private sector, contracting out to civil society can make unrealistic demands of weak government for regulation and the management of contracts. When competitive tendering is involved, it can also lead to civil society providers refusing to co-operate or to share information. Furthermore, aid can undermine advocacy activity by civil society, which is critical in holding rich countries and governments to account.

Don't duplicate, integrate

Civil society can play a key role in providing essential services in poor countries. To maximise efficiency, equity, and access, existing provision by non-state providers, such as for example the churches in Africa, should be integrated into a publicly-led system, but with the NSPs retaining their autonomy. This has been done successfully in Uganda, where the government has given block grants to church providers and has involved them in the overall national plan for health services. Likewise, NGOs in Angola are building essential services as well as the government capacity to run them (see Box 6).

Box 6: NGOs working with governments — building services in Angola

Oxfam NOVIB and its partner Development Workshop are working with local communities and local government to improve essential services in Luanda, Angola. Communities and the municipal administration of Cacuaco drew up agreements to build new schools, employ teachers, and rehabilitate health clinics. The communities are financially and technically supported to plan services and to make their needs and demands heard, while the municipal authority contributes finance, teaching materials, and medicines, and employs new teachers and health workers.

Government staff are closely involved in the process, so that the services developed in partnership with communities can be integrated into the public system. So far, 2,145 children have benefited from improved teaching and learning conditions, and the clinic in Cazenga district now sees 60 patients a day.

Source: Oxfam NOVIB

Stealing staff from poor countries

'They come back every year, and every time they come, we lose dozens of teachers.'
Avril Crawford, President of the Guyana Teachers' Union.

'*They*' are the British recruiters on their annual visit to Guyana to meet teachers replying to their advertisements for applicants to teach in the UK.[169]

Some rich countries are adding insult to injury by actively recruiting health workers and teachers from poor countries to prop up their own public services. One in four doctors in Canada and the USA is from overseas. While the UK government spends £100 million to top up health worker salaries in Malawi, it simultaneously recruits nearly one-third of the doctors in the UK health service from overseas — many from Malawi and other English-speaking African countries. This compares with only 5 per cent in Germany and France.[170]

With the cost of training a general practice doctor estimated at $60,000 and that of training a medical auxiliary at $12,000, the African Union estimates that low-income countries subsidise high-income countries to the tune of $500 million a year through the loss of their health workers. This problem is getting worse, especially in the case of nurses.[171] In the UK during the 1990s there was a huge upsurge in the numbers of African nurses registering for work. There are now more Indian doctors per thousand people in the USA than there are in India.[172] Of the 489 students who graduated from the Ghana Medical School between 1986 and 1995, 61 per cent have left Ghana — with more than half of them going to the UK and one-third to the USA.[173]

The African Union estimates that low-income countries subsidise high-income countries to the tune of $500 million a year through the loss of their health workers.

People in developing countries have the right to travel and to work in other countries, but they also have the right to decent pay and conditions in their own country. A global response to the human resources crisis is needed, in which rich countries address the causes of the workforce crisis in their own public services.

Box 7: Take, take, take

The US government has predicted that the country's shortfall of nurses will rise to 800,000 by 2020. Yet far from training more nurses, the United States Senate is instead choosing to fill this gap with nurses from abroad, passing legislation to remove the limit on the number of nurses who can immigrate to the USA. This is despite the fact that the number of applicants to American nursing colleges greatly exceeds the number of places. Hardest hit is likely to be the Philippines, where 80 per cent of government doctors are busy retraining as nurses in order to secure a green card, according to a survey by Dr. Galvez Tan, at the University of the Philippines. '*I plead for justice,*' he said, '*There has to be give and take, not just take, take, take by the United States.*'[174]

Rich countries still falling short on aid

Rich countries are failing to give enough aid, or to give it in a way that supports governments and public services. What is needed is large amounts of long-term, predictable funding — and rich countries promised to deliver more aid in this form in Paris in early 2005.[175] Instead what they give is far too little aid, which is poorly co-ordinated and scattered across fragmented projects.

Failing to deliver enough, or in the right ways

2005 saw unprecedented pressure put on rich country leaders to increase aid, and a number of new commitments were made. Most notably, European nations collectively promised to increase aid by $40 billion by 2010 and to reach the UN target of giving aid worth 0.7 per cent of their national income by 2015. But this still falls far short of what is needed and, one year on, the underlying trend in countries such as Germany makes even these promises look fragile.[176]

Back in 1995, rich country governments promised to channel 20 per cent of their aid into basic services. By 2004 only Denmark and Ireland had lived up to their pledge; the vast majority of countries were not even close (see Figure 12). These statistics[177] may underestimate the amount given to basic services by rich countries that channel much of their aid directly to governments through 'budget support'. But this is itself a symptom of poor donor reporting of aid to essential services, which needs to improve so that rich countries' commitment to this crucial sector can be monitored.

A recent econometric study of 75 developing countries found that, in some, low and volatile levels of aid explained the slow progress in reducing child deaths.

Furthermore, the volatility of aid is crippling social spending: the money given does not match what was promised and is erratically disbursed, making it hard for recipient governments to pay salaries on time, retain skilled workers, or hire new ones. A recent econometric study of 75 developing countries found that, in some, low and volatile levels of aid explained the slow progress in reducing child deaths.[178]

Aid for water and sanitation needs to double from $14 billion to $30 billion a year, to halve the number of people without access by 2015. But aid for this sector has actually fallen by $1 billion since the early 1990s. Furthermore, it is dominated by a handful of large, urban projects in a few middle-income countries,[179] despite the huge need for investments in rural and peri-urban areas in poor countries.

The Global Fund to fight AIDS, TB and Malaria has so far made grants to 127 countries and will help put 1.8 million people on life-saving treatment for HIV/AIDS — providing it gets the funding its been promised.[180] But the scale of the problem is far greater even than this: around 40 million people worldwide are now infected with HIV, 95 per cent of whom live in developing countries.[181] The Global Fund could do much more, but since it is resourced by *ad hoc* and voluntary contributions from rich countries, it is very difficult for it to scale up services on a sustained basis. In 2005, rich countries held a series of meetings to try to forge a predictable system for replenishing the Fund's finances but, despite enthusiastic statements, the financial commitments for 2006/07 amounted to only $3.7 billion, just over half of the $7.1 billion requested.[182]

There is also a problem in that the Fund is focused on the three killer diseases of AIDS, TB, and malaria and not on strengthening health systems in general. The same applies to many other health interventions by aid donors; overall, just 20 per cent of health financing goes towards the general development of health systems, including health worker salaries.

Figure 12: Broken promises on funding for essential services

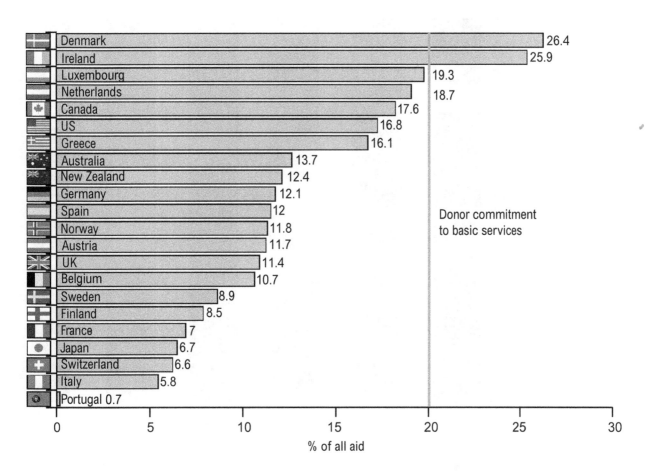

(Source: OECD/DAC 2005)

Aid to education has increased, but UNESCO estimates that a further $17 billion is needed annually to get the remaining 100 million children worldwide into primary school, and to teach illiterate women to read and write. Rich countries set up the Education For All Fast Track Initiative in 2002 and promised aid to every country that produced a good education plan. To date, 37 developing country governments have submitted such plans, but only 16 have received any funding; the funding gap facing even these countries is $430 million. Senior staff at the World Bank have rightly been embarrassed by the shortfall.[183]

Figure 13: Governments taking action, aid donors falling short

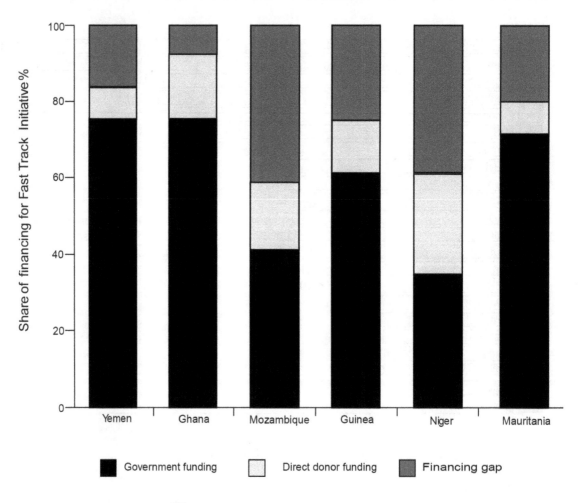

(Source: FTI Secretariat 2005)[184]

Dragging debt

Low levels of aid are exacerbated by the burden of debt. Given the fanfare surrounding the G8's announcements of debt cancellation in 2005, one would be forgiven for thinking that the crisis had finally passed. Not so. Certainly some countries have benefited from the G8's decisions: Zambia, for example, has had all its debts to the IMF cancelled, and this has released vital resources for recruiting more teachers and health workers.[185] But many of the poorest countries, such as Kenya and Bangladesh, have yet to see cancellations, and altogether only 17 countries have had their debts to the IMF and the World Bank written off (although this could rise to 40 over the coming years). African countries have had their debts to the African Development Bank cancelled, but other regional banks, such as the Inter-American Development Bank, have failed to follow suit, leaving countries such as Nicaragua still saddled with major debts. Oxfam and others calculate that more than 60 countries need debt cancellation in order to release the money they need to reach the Millennium Development Goals.

IMF conditions restrict recruitment

'The IMF needs a human face. They should see the children in Africa who are not going to school and start from there with their policies.'
Roy Mwaba, National Union of Teachers, Zambia

IMF policies present massive obstacles for poor countries trying to employ more teachers and health workers. The IMF lends money to poor countries under strict condition that they pursue 'sound' economic policies. If the IMF pulls out, the rich countries will follow. While the IMF is right that countries should manage their economies carefully, its overly rigid stance on public spending is incompatible with achieving the Millennium Development Goals on health, education, and water and sanitation. In Kenya 60,000 teachers are needed to cope with thousands of extra pupils who started coming to school after tuition fees were abolished. But the IMF target to reduce Kenya's public sector wage bill from 8.5 per cent to 7.2 per cent of GDP by 2007 means that teacher numbers have been frozen at their 1998 level.[186]

The IMF's overly rigid stance on public spending is incompatible with achieving the MDGs on health, education, and water and sanitation.

Zambia faces similar constraints. Jennifer Chiwela of the National Education Coalition is frustrated by the contradictions: *'The Education Fast Track Initiative was supposed to help really vulnerable communities do something about their teacher–pupil ratio. But then the IMF and the World Bank said you couldn't go beyond a certain number of teachers. So on the one hand you are setting goals and on the other hand you are creating restrictions which prevent the government from achieving those goals.'*

Why is the IMF standing in the way? It continues to work from a narrow monetarist perspective, which prioritises tight targets on inflation and fiscal deficit over public spending.
At the same time it points to the volatility and unpredictability of aid, and to the potentially negative economic effects caused by large aid inflows. As Box 8 explains, there is good reason for the careful handling of sudden surges of aid, but the appropriate response is better management, not less aid.

Box 8: Dutch disease, or 'Is aid bad for you?'

Attaining the MDGs will require a substantial increase in aid to low-income counties, but the IMF believes that large aid inflows cause economic problems in recipient countries, such as rising inflation, appreciation of the exchange rate, and knock-on effects that undermine a country's economic competitiveness — a syndrome known as 'Dutch disease'.[187]

The fear of Dutch disease, however, seems to be far greater than any evidence that it is actually happening. A recent survey for the IMF of aid in seven countries found little evidence that large scale-ups in aid had actually caused Dutch disease, partly because developing country governments were already used to dealing with the manifold effects of volatile and unpredictable aid.[188]

The implications are that recipient governments need to handle aid increases carefully, as some countries are already doing e.g. by authorising government spending only on aid actually received (Tanzania) or by adjusting aid predictions according to past donor performance (Uganda). And it is imperative for rich countries to improve the reliability and predictability of aid so that it can be used more effectively. Meanwhile scaremongering about the possible future impact of increasing aid when rich countries are already failing to live up to their existing aid commitments is not conducive to meeting the MDGs.

Despite some small changes in recent years, the IMF has not done nearly enough to change the way it works in poor countries in order to make a positive contribution to achieving the MDGs; instead, it often acts as a block to progress. Given this, it is not at all clear that the IMF should continue to play a role in low-income countries. What is clear is that it should certainly not continue in its role as as a 'gatekeeper' for foreign aid.

Failing to co-ordinate means that less gets done

Rich countries are undermining the value of the money they give because it is poorly co-ordinated and is focused on technical assistance and projects. When rich countries met in Rome in 2003 they agreed that, to improve clarity and predictability, they should share a single framework for the procedures and conditionalities of giving aid.[189] Yet a recent OECD survey of 14 developing countries found only three cases where conditionality was streamlined in the health sector, four cases in education, and two cases in water and sanitation.

Angola and DR Congo have each been required to set up four separate HIV/AIDS 'co-ordinating' bodies.

In health the situation is getting worse. The large number of 'vertical' health initiatives is increasing transaction costs, duplicating and undermining health delivery, distorting health priorities, and undermining sector-wide planning. Angola and DR Congo have each been required to set up four separate HIV/AIDS 'co-ordinating' bodies.[190] According to one donor representative in Ethiopia, discussing the various international initiatives to prevent communicable diseases such as HIV/AIDS, malaria, and tuberculosis: *'The Global Fund, PEPFAR, and EMSAP [Ethiopian Multi-Sectoral AIDS Project] are not integrated. From my perspective the benefits are less than the side-effects — disjointed funds waste money, time, and energy.'*[191]

Table 1: Aid that is not co-ordinated does not get used

Country	Utilisation rate of aid for water	
	Government funding	Donor funding
Ethiopia	106%	46%
Ghana	105%	54%
Uganda	65%	44%

(Source: WaterAid 2004)

When there are too many aid sources, with separate reporting demands, money goes unused. Public funding is often preferred even where it is less or late, because it is easier to use (see Table 1). And, as one district assembly chief executive in Ghana explained, '*Most districts are dealing with a variety of rich countries. They all have separate requirements, so the district has up to 20 different bank accounts and I have to write over 200 reports a year.*'[192]

Hung up on technical assistance

Some technical assistance (TA) — such as training, scholarships, studies, and technical advisers — is useful and necessary. But rich countries that spend most of their aid on TA are spending too much money on international consultants (see Table 2). As much as 70 per cent of aid for education is spent on TA,[193] but in fact 70 per cent of the costs of education consist of salaries.[194] In some countries, 100 days of consultancy bills cost the same as paying 100 teachers' salaries for a year or keeping 5,000 children in school.[195] A study of TA in Mozambique found that rich countries were spending a total of $350 million per year on 3,500 technical experts, while 100,000 Mozambican public sector workers were paid a total of just $74 million. The report proposed reallocating some of the TA bill towards local public sector salaries, which would mean 1,000 fewer foreign experts, but the idea was never implemented.[196]

In some countries, 100 days of consultancy bills cost the same as paying 100 teachers' salaries for a year or keeping 5,000 children in school.

According to a senior technical adviser at the Ministry of Health in Malawi: '*Rich countries are scared. They don't mind putting $100 million into building roads. But you say to them "Excuse me sir, we have the best engineer, but we need $100 a month to top up his salary to keep him on." "Impossible," they say, "it can't be done." But they bring in an expert from overseas at $1,000 a day.*'[197]

Aid for projects is also often 'tied' to buying goods and services from the donor country. For example, Spanish aid for constructing a hospital in Nicaragua was tied to buying equipment from Spain. According to the head of the Ministry of Health in San Juan de Dios, '*The equipment was overvalued. It could have been bought from other countries for half the price*'.[198]

Table 2: Highly technical — rich countries that spend over 75 per cent of aid on technical assistance (TA)

Education	% TA	Health	% TA	Water and sanitation	% TA
USA	100	Portugal	98	USA	83
Greece	98	USA	90	Japan	76
Portugal	96	France	84	Netherlands	74
Belgium	95	Australia	81		
Austria	95	Belgium	78		
Germany	94				
Australia	90				
New Zealand	87				
France	87				
Netherlands	82				
Italy	81				
Spain	76				

(Source: OECD/DAC database, December 2005)

Focused on projects, not public systems

The best way for rich countries to help build public services is to put aid into national budget support, as progress in Uganda and Tanzania has shown. Yet less than 5 per cent of bilateral aid was delivered in this way in 2001.[199] The rest went into specific projects. These are useful for piloting new approaches and for one-off interventions, but projects tend to fund investment goods (infrastructure, vehicles, and training) and steer well clear of covering the running costs desperately needed by public systems (salaries, supplies, textbooks, and drugs).

Some rich country governments are making good progress in providing more of their aid through budget support, but it remains a small proportion (less than one-tenth) of their total aid spending (see Figure 14).

Figure 14: Some rich countries are progressing on budget support, most could do more

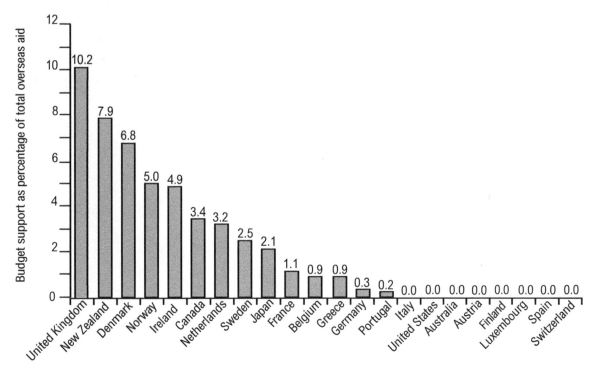

(Source: OECD/DAC online database, May 2006)

Asset-stripping public services

People are an organisation's greatest asset. But when donor projects run parallel to public systems, they compete for — and typically win — the best staff. Ethiopia's Ministry of Health has lost many technical staff to consultancies financed by the Global Fund, where salaries are typically three times higher.[200] Malawi's community-based health services are losing health workers who are retraining as HIV/AIDS counsellors, an area for which there is more funding.[201] In Afghanistan, where rich countries fund international NGOs to deliver the national health-care programme, highly skilled Afghani doctors and nurses are leaving their profession altogether for better-paid jobs as drivers and interpreters in those NGOs. Youssouf Hadeira, a planner in the Ministry of Education in Mali, is faced with the same problem: *'We lose government employees every day to NGOs who offer them better working conditions.'*

Conclusion

Rich countries are crucial partners in helping developing countries to meet the MDGs. But their support is undermined when aid is poorly co-ordinated and concentrated in a patchwork of projects, and when they push for privatisation instead of supporting measures that actually work. Rich countries should co-ordinate their efforts around national plans; build the capacity of government departments to plan, manage, and deliver essential services effectively; and provide the long-term, predictable, and sustainable finance needed to back this up.

5

Time to deliver:
how developing countries and rich country governments can build effective public services

LUUM!
CHAMA CHA MAEN?
SIASA
HATUTAKI SIAS
MWENYE SIASA
CHAMA CHA S

5

Time to deliver: how developing countries and rich country governments can build effective public services

What developing countries need to do

Getting the politics right

> '*I am happy to say that [my] government has kept its promise of providing free and compulsory primary education... [and] remains committed to universal primary education by 2015.*'
> President Kibaki of Kenya, in the State Opening of Parliament, 2003

The Kenyan government is better known for its problems (most recently concerning corruption) than its successes, but 11-year-old John Nzomo is one of the many thousands of Kenyans to benefit from President Kibaki's commitment to education. In the days when there were fees for children attending primary school, his parents could not afford them, so he had to drop out. But in January 2003, the newly-elected president held to one of his core manifesto promises to make primary education free. Since then, John — and 1.2 million more Kenyan children, many of them girls — have been going to school. '*It was a miracle for us that free primary education came,*' said his mother. '*Otherwise, John would still be at home.*'[202]

Kenya's education crisis is not yet over, but the political commitment to free primary education is a watershed. It is changing people's perception of education: from a privilege for the wealthy into a right for all. There are benefits for democracy too: putting education at the heart of political campaigning has moved Kenya another step away from ethnicity-based politics, towards politics based on national development concerns and the fight against poverty.

The repeated failure of many governments to fulfil their people's rights to basic education, health care, and water and sanitation has been one of the biggest political scandals in the developing world over the past 25 years. This is clearly demonstrated in the 2005 Social Watch report, which documents how in many countries spending on social services is decreasing whilst inequality increases.[203] Yet in many countries failures to deliver on such fundamentals of the social contract between citizen and state have fallen far down the political agenda. If there is to be success in delivering essential services to poor people, then what has started happening in Kenya must happen across the developing world.

opposite page
Protest march in Kibera, Kenya,
'*We asked for trained teachers from the government, and for a school feeding programme...*
The [government] came to Kibera within a week.
We weren't aware of our power. It's been a great revelation to us. Even the police were saying,
"*This is not a bad march, they are only demanding their rights*"'—
Maurice Odek, Kibera

The first step towards providing essential services for all is getting the politics right. How? Developing country governments need to:

- Shift the political agenda,
- Strive for equity for women,
- Fulfil rights by removing user fees,
- Fight corruption and build accountability, and
- Strengthen public capacity.

Shift the political agenda

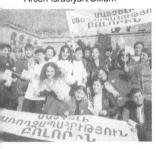

More than 500 people marched through Yerevan, Armenia, calling on the government to make sure that everyone has access to essential health-care services

Political commitment is the key to making services work, and to do this governments must feel the heat. In Kerala state in India and in Sri Lanka, politically-aware citizens demanded services that performed well. A closed clinic generated social protest, and governments were forced to respond. In Mauritius and Barbados, competitive electoral politics drove the state's interest in delivering services. In other high-performing countries, such as Malaysia or, more recently, Uganda and Brazil, national leaders who considered essential services central to national development and unity have played a crucial role. A common thread in all these cases is the compact formed between the state and its citizens: governments delivered essential services, which people came to expect as their right. Building people's expectations is key to getting essential services onto the political agenda, and also makes services harder to dismantle subsequently.

Civil society organisations build expectations and push for change. Across the world, they are getting debates on essential services into the newspapers and onto politicians' lists of priorities. In Kenya the national coalition of education groups, Elimu Yetu (Our Education) played a pivotal role in putting free primary education on the agenda and in keeping it there. WaterAid and Oxfam International are supporting partners in countries across the developing world to get essential services onto the political agenda and to challenge governments to improve their performance.

The Global Campaign for Education is uniting education activists worldwide in publicising the issues and pressurising governments into action. In 2005 the world's biggest ever anti-poverty coalition was formed, the Global Call to Action against Poverty (GCAP). GCAP organised mobilisation and campaigning in 2005 that saw over 36 million people take action in more than 80 countries. All of these actions were united under the symbol of the white band. GCAP has continued into 2006, and has renewed its call to governments both North and South to end poverty. Among GCAP's key demands are quality universal public services for all and an end to privatisation where it causes deprivation and poverty.

As is the case anywhere, the political scene in developing countries is dominated by national elites, who can either drive or block progress on public services. The huge differences in performance on health and education by countries at similar stages of economic development show that some elites are more progressive or more amenable to argument than others.

Agriculturally-based elites tend to be more hostile to public services than urban or industrial groups: they have a vested interest in maintaining a supply of low-skilled, low-paid agricultural labour, and are keen to avoid empowering small farmers who might demand redistribution of their own large and often inefficient farms.[204] The semi-feudal nature of social relations in many rural areas makes large landowners keen to preserve their status. Thankfully, one of the side-effects of urbanisation is the decline of such bastions of reaction.

One recent study of how elites in a number of developing countries regard poverty found a number of causes for optimism.[205] Firstly, elites are increasingly moved by 'positive drivers', such as a belief in national development or national pride and unity, rather than by 'negative drivers' such as fears of disease or revolution. Secondly, they are now more likely to take a 'human resource approach' to national development, accepting that a nation's future depends on the education and health of its people. In the past, elites were often seduced by the glamour of prestige projects such as dams or airports, rather than paying attention to the humdrum business of schools and clinics. Interestingly, surveys have shown strongest elite support for education, more than for health or other public services; it can hardly be a coincidence that in recent decades progress on schools has been faster than that on clinics, taps, or toilets.

Such results underline the benefits of building a dialogue between national elites, social movements, and the international community, and of highlighting the benefits of improving public services as the best use of both tax revenue and aid.

Targeting essential services towards poor people can actually result in them losing out. Rich people are more likely to pay taxes for something that they themselves use.

Paradoxically, targeting essential services towards poor people can actually result in them losing out. Rich people are more likely to pay taxes for something that they themselves use. Targeting particular interventions (free school meals, water subsidies, etc.) at poor people works if it is done in addition to providing essential services universally. But targeting essential services at poor people in place of universal public provision, while it might seem cheaper in the short term, often results in wealthier groups withdrawing financial and political support for public services where they see no benefit to themselves.

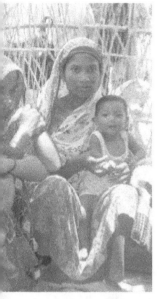

All the village committee members in Gaibandha, Bangladesh, are women. They meet once a week to discuss issues such as personal hygiene, farming, and the positioning of latrines and tube wells.

Strive for equity

Make services work for women

Investing in basic services that support and empower women and girls is crucial — and governments can learn a lot from women's organisations about the best way to make services work for them. How can it be done? By promoting women as workers, supporting women and girls as service users, protecting them from abuse, working with women's organisations, and combining these measures with legal reforms that improve the status and autonomy of women in society.

Promote and retain female staff

When women are at the front-line of delivering services, their presence encourages other women and girls to use those services. In Palestine, where the vast majority of teachers are women, net primary enrolment rates are among the highest in the Middle East and 97 per cent of girls go on to secondary school.[206] Likewise, the presence of female doctors and health workers makes it far more likely that women and girls will come to clinics when they need health or maternal care. Increasing female employment also increases women's financial independence.

Fair wages are an essential first step in bringing women into essential services, but wider support can help them move into public service jobs. The Gambian government, for example, set up a scheme to support young women enrolling in teacher training.[207] Quotas for female teacher recruitment have also been effective.

Support women with welfare payments

Welfare payments that put cash in the hands of women enable them and their children to use services. In South Africa, pensions for low-income individuals are the basis of the government's poverty alleviation programme. These pensions reach over 80 per cent of the elderly population, the majority of whom are women.[208] Despite gaps in coverage, and discrepancies in eligibility between married and single women, the scheme is said to be 'one of the most effective poverty alleviation and redistribution tools — especially in relation to women, who constitute the majority of the poor in South Africa'.[209]

Protect women and girls from abuse

Combating sexual harassment and violence against women and girls is crucial, both for women who use services and for women who deliver them. Governments committed to ending the daily harassment that takes place have formulated protection policies which, combined with public campaigning, can help when the problem is exacerbated by a culture of silence. In Uganda, the Ministry of Education has highlighted the abuse of girls in school, and this has led to the dismissal and even imprisonment of some teachers and male students. When communities are aware of successful legal cases and when the media draw attention to the issue, other girls are encouraged to speak out.[210]

Work at all levels

The best way to make services work for women and girls is by simultaneously working with women's groups, changing laws, and challenging harmful beliefs. When these multiple initiatives are combined, they can result in rapid progress.

- **Working with women's movements.** When governments and women's organisations work together, they can achieve a greater impact than either can working separately. In Brazil, women's organisations working within and outside government ensured that the 1988 Constitution reflected the importance of women's reproductive health.[211] Women's movements have continued to influence public health policy: an integrated women's health programme has been established (Programa de Assistencia a Saude da Mulher — PAISM) and special health services are now available to victims of rape. In Tanzania during the 1990s, the Ministry of Education and Culture worked with the Forum of African Women in Education (FAWE) and with universities to reach out to girls and teachers through workshops, popular media, and drama. The Ministry ran awareness-raising sessions for senior officials and made the school curriculum more relevant to female students.[212]

- **Changing laws.** South Africa's ANC government rewrote the constitution to promote women's equality and rights. The result? Today one in two public servants in South Africa is a woman, and women account for one-third of members of the National Assembly — up from just 3 per cent during the apartheid era.[213] Quotas can work too. In 1992 India made a constitutional amendment that reserved one-third of local government seats for women, and this has given more weight to women's concerns in the political agenda. On average, local councils that have a majority of women spend more on public water facilities and on providing latrines for low-caste groups.[214]

- **Challenging beliefs.** Good interventions go beyond providing services to women: they enable women to empower themselves in the process. Education curricula have a vital role to play in changing perceptions of women's status. India's Total Literacy Campaign, launched by the government in 1988 and implemented by local government administrators with the NGO Bharat Gyun Vigyan Samiti (BGVS), increased adult literacy levels and prompted women participants to begin questioning the social norms constraining their lives.

In Brazil, women's organisations working within and outside government influence public health policy: an integrated women's health programme has been established (Programa de Assistencia a Saude da Mulher — PAISM) and special health services are now available to victims of rape.

Fulfil rights by removing user fees

'In the past in order to access health care you had to have money. If my child was sick, I had to pay 20 pesos to the paediatrician every time we had to see him. We don't have to do that any more. Our medical services are free for everybody. That's a big change.'
Dr. Sandra Pérez, Cuba

Abolishing user fees for primary education and basic health care is one of the most important steps a government can take towards getting the politics of essential services right. Such a step can make a government more directly accountable to its citizens than can any number of public financial management reforms. It signals that access to health care, education, and safe water and sanitation are inalienable human rights, and it puts essential services back in their rightful place at the top of the political agenda. It makes it harder for future governments to backtrack on essential services, once people have got used to sending their children to school and being able to use the local clinic. It is also a powerful catalyst for raising the quality and efficiency of services.

South Africa's new government recognised the barriers that user charges posed to poor people, and so increased the health budget, directed more of it into primary care, and introduced the Free Care Policy for basic health services. This policy resulted in a 20–60 per cent increase in the use of public facilities, especially for child and maternal health. Within two years, 75 per cent of public health workers believed that the policy was successfully preventing death and serious illness among women and children under six years old.[215] This is despite the South African government's inaction over providing universal access to antiretrovirals for people living with HIV/AIDS.

Abolishing user fees in basic education and health care in 20 African countries would save the lives of 250,000 children each year.

Likewise, other African countries have boosted primary education by abolishing school fees. Figure 15 shows the immediate impact this has on getting children into school.

Governments should commit to removing fees for basic health care and education, and rich country governments should fund this process until countries can afford these costs themselves. Recent calculations by Save the Children UK show that abolishing user fees in basic education and health care in 20 African countries would save the lives of 250,000 children each year and cost less than 6 per cent of the $18 billion investment needed to meet the health MDGs.[216]

Figure 15: Abolishing fees gets education on the agenda and kids into school

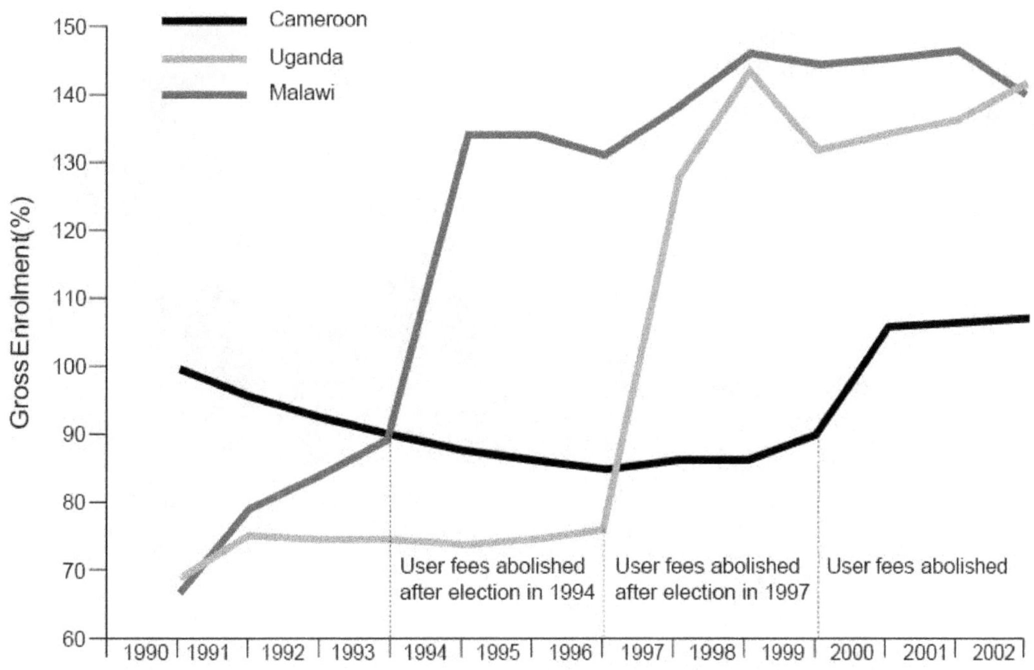

Legend: Cameroon, Uganda, Malawi

Y-axis: Gross Enrolment(%), 60 to 150

X-axis: 1990 to 2002

User fees abolished after election in 1994

User fees abolished after election in 1997

User fees abolished

(Source: World Bank website: http://devdata.worldbank.org/edstats/query/default.htm)

It should be remembered that user fees are just part of a broader issue of how to ensure sustainable, predictable, and adequate financing for public services. Abolishing government fees will exacerbate problems — and even result in the proliferation of informal fees and charges — unless accompanied by a range of other reforms, including increased and better-directed funding. As a minimum, the revenue lost from fees must be replaced so that schools and clinics do not lose out.

Community health insurance[217] is a slightly better alternative to user fees in health services, but is only a short-term stopgap in dealing with underlying financing problems. Such schemes can, however, provide limited financial protection from health crises in the short term, as Oxfam's health programme in the Caucasus shows (see Box 11).

Box 9: Community health insurance — a short-term alternative to user fees

Oxfam GB runs community financing schemes in remote districts of Armenia where public provision is absent or of very low quality. Under the scheme, members pay a small quarterly fee equivalent to about $5 and receive assistance from the village nurse at the health clinic, together with free essential drugs and monthly visits from a doctor. Without the scheme, patients would have to travel to the nearest town and pay upfront to see a doctor and buy drugs.

As Amalia Ohajanyan, a 69-year old patient, explained: *'The scheme has really helped the village. Before, if we had a health problem, we had to go to Kapan. That takes money and time. If we could find a car, we would borrow it, but often it was impossible.'*

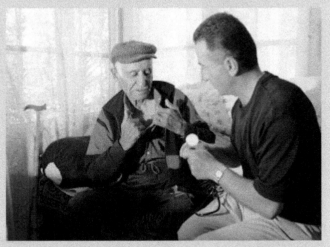

Nurse Nersiyan treats Hovsep Karapetyan, a member of the Oxfam community-based health scheme in Khachik village, Armenia

Toby Adamson/Oxfam

In Uganda, the failure of community health insurance schemes to attract a large membership or to reach poorer groups persuaded the government to abolish user fees in public clinics.

Unfortunately the population coverage of such schemes is low, and they cover only part of the cost of delivering the service and need extensive public subsidy to operate in the long term.[218] For these reasons, Oxfam is working with the government in Armenia so that it can eventually take over the costs and run the health schemes itself. In Uganda, the government experimented with community health insurance schemes in the 1990s, but the failure of the schemes to attract a large membership or to reach poorer groups was one factor that persuaded the government to abolish user fees in public clinics instead.[219]

Subsidise taps and toilets

In water services, unlike in health and education, user fees are needed in order to encourage sustainable use of finite water resources. It is crucial, however, that the structure and affordability of water tariffs are managed in order to achieve equitable access for poor people in urban areas.

- In Porto Alegre, Brazil, water consumption is subsidised, with the first 10,000 litres discounted to the price of 4,000 litres.
- In Uganda, the water utility NWSC provides community water points that are managed by private individuals, where the price of water is publicised at the tap and is much lower than for water provided by private vendors. It also provides cheaper options to poorer consumers, by giving free connection to yard taps for households living within 50 metres of the main pipe.

- In South Africa, the first 6,000 litres of water per month are supplied free (equivalent to 25 litres per person per day), meaning that poor consumers are guaranteed a minimum amount of water.

The exact tariff/fee structure will depend on the country context and needs to be determined by full consultation with both users and providers.

Fight corruption and build accountability

Corruption needs to be fought on a number of different levels. Firstly, at the level of society as a whole. The extent of corruption in public services is primarily a reflection of the society in which those services operate. In countries where the rule of law exists and where there are an ethos of trust and strong accountability mechanisms, there will be far less corruption in services. Strong public education services can play an important role in instilling in children a culture of trust, honesty, and respect for the rule of law. So can public awareness campaigns. In Uganda, Oxfam has supported the anti-corruption coalition, which has sought to draw attention to the harmful effects of corruption through public campaigning.

Corruption also needs to be tackled at the political level. If the problem is to be successfully addressed, it has to become politically impossible for leaders or elites to abuse public resources for their own private gain. In many countries, multi-party democracy and the emergence of civil society and a free press are proving to be key building blocks in the fight against corruption. Scandals uncovered recently by the press in Costa Rica and Kenya, for example, have led to the prosecution of key senior officials.

Government and business leaders must signal their intolerance of corruption and their commitment to accountability. In Uganda, one of the first actions taken by the CEO of the National Water and Sewerage Corporation before the successful reform of the organisation was to publish his own phone number in the press, so that people could complain to him directly about the quality of the service they received.[220] In Recife in Brazil, the mayor organised city-wide reviews of services with citizen groups to discuss how the performance of municipal utilities could be improved.[221] Parliaments are also increasingly scrutinising government, often with assistance from civil society.

Government and business leaders must signal their commitment to accountability. In Recife, the mayor organised city-wide reviews of services with citizen groups.

Civil society itself is playing an increasingly important and vocal role in holding political leaders to account, tracking government expenditures on essential services and highlighting instances where money is going missing. In Georgia, for example, Oxfam supports the Georgian Young Economists organisation in analysing the government budget and in publishing its findings. In Sierra Leone, civil society groups found that 30 per cent of school pupils had not received textbooks.

Workers in the public sector must be seen as part of the solution, not just as the problem.[222] In many cases, improved salaries, status, and conditions have helped to reduce corruption. This approach is especially effective when combined with the introduction of codes of conduct and strengthened accountability mechanisms.

In Cambodia and the Czech Republic, salary top-ups for health workers, combined with commitments to codes of ethical good practice, led to a decline in informal bribe payments and greater access to health services by poor people.[223] Cameroon, Finland, and Guatemala have increased transparency in public procurement — one of the biggest sources of corruption. Brazil and Georgia have improved the capacity of their judiciaries to tackle corruption cases and have introduced codes of conduct. Rules to prevent conflicts of interest in public office have been implemented in New Zealand and Panama.[224]

To combat corruption there must be investment in other key services, not least the legal system and the audit functions of government.

To combat corruption in services such as health and education, there must be investment in other key services, not least the legal system and the audit functions of government. In Malawi, for instance, there are just 195 lawyers for 11 million people.[225] Public administrators, managers, and regulators, though much maligned, need to be increased in number and need to be better resourced. Unions and professional associations play an important role as partners in developing professional standards and engaging workers in improving services.

Citizens themselves also need to be able, wherever possible, to directly scrutinise providers of services and to hold them to account. In Zambia, the Zambia Reflect Network is involving local communities in monitoring finances in schools. Gina Fundafunda is its chairperson: '*We are involving communities in seeing that schools are run properly. We are training people to check what happens to the money once it has been allocated to the school — is it actually getting to where it's meant to? — so that the communities are able to say, "What do we need here, how do we help?".*'

However, such mechanisms are very time-consuming and cannot take the place of formal accountability mechanisms, such as parliaments and professional codes of conduct. Ultimately there is no magic answer to corruption: it is a society-wide problem that affects both the public and private sectors, and rich and poor countries alike. It has to be tackled at the societal, political, and technical levels, and governments, civil society, parliaments, citizens, and rich country aid donors all have critical roles to play.

Institutionalise citizen representation

The role of citizen oversight needs to be institutionalised, making people daily participants in the improvement of the services they use — and not merely as consumers with financial power, as this would exclude those denied an effective voice by their lack of cash. In practice, citizens need a formally recognised role in public oversight institutions, a right to register complaints and refer to a higher body, and the right to review official information.

In Zambia and Baluchistan, Pakistan the involvement of parent-teacher committees in the management and monitoring of schools has improved the quality and efficiency of school performance.[226] The Swedish government is working with the Ministry of Health and Family Welfare in Bangladesh to set up a Health Service Users Forum at national level, linked to community- and district-level monitoring groups.[227] Ombudsmen are a useful means of building citizens' views and complaints into health services, and Oxfam has instigated initiatives of this kind in Armenia and Georgia, along with its support to public clinics. WaterAid has set up feedback mechanisms between water user groups and local governments in Nepal, India, Bangladesh, Ghana, and Ethiopia.[228]

Strengthen public capacity

'In the past, when I was a student, teachers were respected. Respect for teachers declined after the 1980s when teachers' salaries became much lower. Parents do not respect teachers at all, and once a student said to one of our teachers, "Why do you waste your time teaching when you earn so little?".'
Male teacher, Mwanza, Tanzania[230]

Building a public service ethos

The countries that have been successful have built an ethos of public service, in which public sector workers are encouraged to take pride in their contribution to the nation and to society, and society in turn is urged to grant them status and respect. Public sector workers need to be supported both to do their job and to engage in the continual improvement of service provision. In the Philippines, for example, the union PSLINK mobilised its members to monitor drug procurement and delivery of school textbooks, and also provides legal protection for members who expose corruption.[231]

In the Philippines, the union PSLINK mobilised its members to monitor drug procurement and delivery of school textbooks.

The majority of health workers are dedicated professionals trying to cope in difficult and frustrating environments. But the way workers are treated by the public systems in which they work influences the way that they in turn treat the people who use their services. Poor pay, low status, and low morale cause poor performance and encourage corrupt behaviour in the public sector. Countries that have succeeded in tackling these problems have improved the status and remuneration of workers, while simultaneously insisting on performance improvements and strengthened accountability mechanisms.

The Ugandan public water utility NWSC has created an environment of innovation, problem solving, accountability, and customer focus through a performance contract agreed with the government, which specifies performance targets and social obligations. At the same time, NWSC has managerial autonomy from the government and has developed clear performance agreements with its staff, who are then rewarded for progress.[232]

Evidence shows that higher salaries for health workers are linked to reductions in bribe-taking and informal payments.

Higher pay and performance incentives help. Evidence from Poland, Cambodia, and the Czech Republic shows that higher salaries for health workers are linked to reductions in bribe-taking and informal payments.[233] In Bangladesh, India, and Nepal, codes of conduct have had a significant positive impact on the commitment, professional behaviour, and performance of teachers and staff and have contributed to a reduction in teacher absenteeism.[234]

Building partnerships between neighbouring public water and sanitation utilities is helping to improve performance and the public service ethos in many countries, by sharing technical and managerial know-how. These so-called Public–Public Partnerships (or PuPs) already exist in some corners of the world — for example, NWSC in Uganda is providing assistance and advice to Tanzania's DAWASCO to improve its billing and collection systems, while in India the Bangalore Water Supply and Sewerage Board is set to provide assistance to the Delhi Jal Board for leakage control. More support could be provided to expand these Public–Public Partnerships.

Tackling the workforce crisis is possible — and cost-effective

Drastically scaling up the numbers of teachers and health workers is a huge task that requires strategic, co-ordinated planning between governments from both poor and rich countries. Governments need to produce and implement strategic workforce plans that specify how many and which types of workers are needed and how much this will cost. Countries which have successfully scaled up health and education services have included workforce planning as part of the process from the outset. For example, in Botswana the Ministry of Health has developed a database of its current health workforce and its projected needs, which it links to its five-year National Development Plans.[235]

In the health sector, community and informal health workers can help to plug a critical gap in health systems, providing they are well integrated into the health system. Community-based barefoot doctors and nurses have played a vital part in expanding services in successful countries, as have temporary or partly-trained teachers. However, this strategy does not work when it is used to undermine the existing profession. Governments should first bring into the workforce any trained but unemployed public service workers or retired professionals, and seek to attract back any trained staff who have moved to other jobs. If there is still a gap, then (in consultation with unions) emergency measures can be taken to increase numbers, but the aim should be to give new recruits opportunities to become fully professional within a few years.

In water supply, scaling up will require better information on gaps in supply, more inclusive and participatory planning and close co-operation with communities to sustain services. In Tanzania the legal recognition of community-owned water service organisations made it easier for local governments to help with repairs and maintenance and with monitoring water quality.[236] Scaling up sanitation requires sustained public campaigning about hand-washing and healthy behaviour and subsidies for latrine construction.

Improving pay and conditions

Pay on its own does not always increase motivation, but it is the first priority where earnings are currently too low to meet the cost of living, as has been demonstrated by countries that have successfully tackled worker shortages. Better pay needs to be matched with better conditions. For most teachers, housing is a major issue, and one that will have to be addressed if governments are to persuade more teachers to work in rural areas. This applies especially to women teachers, whose physical security and ability to care for their families can be put at risk by working in isolated rural locations.

Pay on its own does not always increase motivation, but it is the first priority where earnings are currently too low to meet the cost of living.

Box 11: Government-led emergency human resources programme — Malawi

'My message to rich countries? We would love to save our people. We don't want to go abroad for the money. Home is the base.'
Rosemary Bilesi, nursing officer, Dowa District Hospital, Malawi

'The impact of the salary top-up? In 2003, resignations of nurses were at one or even two a week. It was shocking. Since we introduced incentives, including the locum system, we've somehow stemmed it to one or two a month.'
Dr. Damison Kathyola, director of Kamuzu Central Hospital, Lilongwe

'The top-ups and locum system have helped. At least we can receive additional nurses and clinicians from other hospitals who come for relief duties. Before, maternal mortality was a big problem and nurses had no time to monitor pregnant women. So now pregnant women are being served better.'
Moses Ngwira, deputy district health officer and clinical officer in Dowa District Hospital

The health worker crisis in Malawi is chronic — but the government is starting to turn the situation around by working in partnership with rich country aid donors to build public services.

Decades of low pay, poor working conditions, and under-funding have undermined the public health system and have led to a chronic shortage of nurses and doctors. Vacancies in nursing posts are running at over 60 per cent, and four of Malawi's districts have no doctors at all. Existing staff are leaving the public health system to work for civil society organisations or private hospitals, or even deserting the health sector altogether.

The UK government has been working closely with Malawi's Ministry of Health to tackle the country's severe human resources problems. In 2004 the Ministry produced a six-year human resources relief programme, which is 90 per cent funded by the UK and the Global Fund. The assistance is funding:

- a 50 per cent increase in the salaries of 5,400 existing front-line health workers;

- the recruitment of 700 new health staff, with a planned doubling of health workers in six years through expansion and improvement of training schools and trainers; and

- the plugging of critical gaps with expatriate volunteers: 20 doctors from the UK NGO Voluntary Services Overseas (VSO) and 18 specialists have already arrived, while more Malawians are being trained.

Even though the programme has been criticised for bypassing health unions, it is already having an impact. Funds only started being released in April 2005, but there are early indications from hospitals of a dramatic reduction in the outflow of nurses.

Sources: DFID personal communication and DFID 2004

Build government capacity to plan and manage systems

The abolition of user fees in the Ugandan health system was accompanied by vital investments in the system's capacity. A comprehensive plan for the health sector was drawn up and management capacity was strengthened. The planning and budget system was improved to even out regional financing disparities and to improve the flow of funds to front-line facilities. Funds were dispersed more rapidly and the payroll was computerised to pay health workers' salaries more quickly. A quarterly monitoring system was set up to measure the performance of spending at the district level. The role of non-state health providers was examined, and a new system of grant financing was set up to fund the recurrent costs of mission hospitals providing care in rural areas.

Increasingly, civil society groups and parliaments are being included in planning processes. The Ugandan government plan, for example, was heavily influenced by the findings of the Ugandan Participatory Poverty Assessment Project (UPPAP), previously carried out in collaboration with Ugandan civil society groups. Such groups also have a key role to play in publicising progress and in holding governments to account when they fail to deliver.

Unfortunately the Ugandan experience is the exception rather than the rule. If services are to be expanded, then governments must invest in competent managers and planners to produce and implement clearly costed plans. Budget disbursement and financial management procedures need to be strengthened to get money to the right people and the right places at the right time. Clear workforce strategies are needed to plan the numbers of employees that will be needed over the long term.

Clear workforce strategies are needed to plan the numbers of employees that will be needed over the long term.

A number of governments have developed plans of this nature. School enrolments in Bogotá, Colombia increased by nearly 40 per cent, while costs increased by only half as much, thanks to a new information system and negotiations with teacher unions that deployed teachers where they were needed and eliminated 'ghost' teachers. Ethiopia and Brazil overcame regional disparities in education funding by using national revenue to cross-subsidise schools in poorer areas.[237]

In the water sector, separating utilities from political interference and making them financially autonomous has been key to improving performance. Publicly-owned utilities in Uganda, Porto Alegre in Brazil, and Penang in Malaysia have shown that combining a commercial ethos with social obligations can improve both efficiency and equity in water and sanitation supply, and that contracting in private providers for some operations — as opposed to full privatisation — can be useful.

In rural areas too, improvements in local government planning can help to expand services, and do it more equitably. In Nigeria, Ghana, and Nepal, for example, WaterAid and partners have worked to strengthen local government planning capacity, using improved information and public consultations to produce local water development plans. These plans help local authorities to negotiate for more resources from central government and strengthen citizens' ability to hold local governments to account.

Improve the effectiveness and progressiveness of tax collection

Taxes are the cornerstone of health and education funding, so improvements are urgently needed. As a proportion of GDP, tax collection in poor countries is less than half that in rich countries.[238] This is largely because elites have proved adept both at evading tax and ensuring that tax laws are lenient, should they choose to pay. Efforts to expand tax revenue in many countries in recent years have involved an increase in indirect taxation (such as VAT and sales taxes) but, without significant exemptions, such measures can shift a greater burden of taxation onto poor people. Nevertheless, progress is possible. South Africa has recently increased its tax take while at the same time reducing income tax rates, by imposing heavy penalties on tax fraudsters.

One under-researched impact of the drive for trade liberalisation is a serious fall in government revenue from import taxes, often on luxury goods, which are particularly important in low-income countries. A 2005 IMF study found that broader tax reforms have allowed poor country governments to make up only 30 per cent of the revenue lost through tariff cuts.[239]

What rich countries need to do

The best way for rich countries to help achieve the MDGs is to support developing country governments and peoples in implementing the kinds of measures outlined above. Rich countries need to support public systems and public capacity. They must stop bypassing and undermining governments by pushing for the expansion of private service provision, and instead must provide long-term, predictable financing for the salaries and running costs of public systems, whether or not they choose to involve NSPs or the private sector in their delivery.

As the case of Uganda shows, sector and budget support programmes are best suited to funding a national expansion of social services, rather than providing support for specific projects, which may take years to design and which are often a highly inefficient form of finance.[240] A recent independent evaluation of budget support in seven developing countries found that, provided governments have the political will, budget support can encourage spending on health and education, make governments' planning and spending more transparent and accountable, and strengthen their relationships with aid providers.[241]

In Tanzania, where general budget support accounts for about 36 per cent of all aid flows, external funds and policy dialogue at the highest levels have facilitated an expansion in the financing and provision of education and health services.[242] Budget support will not be appropriate in all countries. It requires levels of accountability, efficiency, and transparency which may be lacking in some countries. In these cases projects can be a useful way of innovating new approaches and, indeed, governments in countries that are not highly dependent on aid, such as India, may prefer project aid.

In the health sector, most donors need to make a step-change in the way they think and act, moving from disease-specific and vertical interventions that drain government capacity to a system-wide approach that strengthens capacity to deliver. The Red Cross took this approach in Serbia, where it was initially called on to address the health needs of refugees. Rather than building separate clinics, the organisation decided to strengthen the entire primary health-care system at the district level. A new funding system for clinics was designed, the district IT system was updated, and health workers were trained. The result? Improved access to health care for the whole district — and the government has since taken over many of the reforms, improving its own ability to provide health care in the long term.[243]

Rich country governments can use aid to improve accountability. In Malawi — seen as a high-risk country under its previous government, due to endemic corruption — donors are now financing the salaries of health workers. They are also working with the government to build strong institutions: more accountants are being hired to conduct independent financial and procurement audits and technical advisors are mentoring senior Malawian civil servants.[244]

Many important decisions and opportunities arise at local level. Box 12 shows how rich country governments and civil society organisations can work directly with different tiers of government in developing countries to achieve the MDGs.

Most donors need to make a step-change in the way they think and act, moving from disease-specific and vertical interventions to a system-wide approach that strengthens capacity to deliver.

Box 12: How to support local government and build planning capacity

WaterAid has developed a new set of initiatives to strengthen the capacity of local governments in Nigeria, Ghana, Burkina Faso, Mali, and Nepal. The process is funded primarily by WaterAid, which also provides technical assistance support to the local government, while local NGOs facilitate public participation processes. The 'Localising MDG Initiative' works with existing structures of government agencies and elected government officials to:

- build the information base so that local governments can determine the best strategic use of their investments for the whole decade up to 2015;

- strengthen team work between government departments and community groups/leaders by sharing information and facilitating discussions on plans; and

- develop a local service plan agreed by officials and community leaders. This plan then becomes the basis for the local government's requests for funding from central government.

Source: WaterAid (2005b)

Governments and rich country aid donors need to ensure that the aid relationship does not squeeze out policy dialogue with civil society at the local level. Reliance on aid must not become an impediment to democracy.

Tackle the demand side of the brain drain

> *'I want to go back, but I need something to supplement my income because I know the Malawian nursing salary is not going to be enough for me to live on and provide for my children. That is the only thing that is keeping me here. So I am here to save money so that I can return to work as a nurse in Malawi.'*
>
> Mary Ntata, a Malawian nurse who came to the UK for medical training

Teachers and nurses have a right to migrate, but people in poor countries also have a right to expect publicly-trained professionals to stay and work in their home country for a number of years after graduation. A global response to the human resources crisis is needed. Although there can be benefits for developing countries from migration, particularly of low-skilled workers (e.g. through remittance flows), rich countries must address the causes of the workforce crisis in their own public services, and avoid cherry picking the skilled workers that developing countries so desperately need. Ethical codes of practice for recruiting countries have been tried, with some success. For example, the United Kingdom's ethical recruitment code has halted the increase in recruitment of overseas nurses in the National Health Service, though most private agencies do not apply the code.

Countries receiving essential workers can invest in the institutions of those sending them, as a form of restitution. A global education reinvestment fund has also been suggested, to accelerate the training of health professionals in developing countries by supporting public efforts and by offering incentives for private investments.

Increase and improve aid and cancel debts

Bangladesh should not have to pay back debt when 50 million of its people live on less than a dollar a day.

While the past five years have seen genuine progress, debt cancellation must be extended to all the countries that need it, if the fight against poverty is to be won. The Jubilee Debt Campaign calculates that over 60 countries will need all of their debts cancelled — and this cancellation must not be undermined by tying it to the implementation of harmful economic policies.

A fair and transparent process must be established, independent of creditors such as the World Bank and the IMF, to judge what debts a poor country can afford to pay. Bangladesh should not have to pay back debt when 50 million of its people live on less than a dollar a day. The process should acknowledge that many debts are illegitimate and should not be paid. South Africa, for example, has spent hundreds of millions of dollars paying back the debts incurred by the racist apartheid regime, money that would be better used in dealing with that system's legacy of poverty and inequality. Jubilee Research estimates that about $11.7 billion of South Africa's current foreign debt comes from interest on apartheid-era loans.

The developing world needs to see far more aid, and to see that aid better spent. Even with the promises made in 2005 at Gleneagles, by 2010 rich countries will only be giving 0.36 per cent of their income in aid — the same proportion as in 1987 and only half the 0.7 per cent target agreed in 1970. Rich countries must increase their aid to 0.7 per cent by 2010 at the latest.

In addition, the money they do give needs to be far better spent. As the example of DFID in Malawi shows, rich countries can have a powerful impact on building public services in poor countries, but not when they waste money on superfluous consultants, or insist that the aid is spent on their own exports, or when they spend too much money on projects instead of systems. In countries where there is clearly a commitment to fight poverty, donors must increase the amount they give directly in support of government plans and budgets. They must co-ordinate more, to minimise the burden on overworked government staff in poor countries. They must also commit for the long term, so that governments can train and pay the massive numbers of new teachers and health workers that are needed. They must expand and fully finance the Education For All Fast Track Initiative and the Global Fund to Fight Aids, TB and Malaria, and ensure that these too support governments and public systems. Finally, they must end, once and for all, the practice of insisting that developing country governments implement harmful economic policies, such as inappropriate privatisation or rapid and indiscriminate trade liberalisation, in order to receive aid.

The IMF monopoly on determining what constitutes 'sound economic policies' should be ended. The IMF should ensure that its advice to developing countries does not undermine efforts to scale up health and education services by placing excessive restrictions on government spending.

Help to get rid of user fees

Given the weight of evidence, the World Bank should be using its considerable influence — not least as the largest health-sector donor in Africa — to actively support the abolition of user fees in health and education. After all, it was the Bank that originally advocated the introduction of fees as part of its structural adjustment programmes in the 1990s. Subsequently in 2003 the Bank disavowed them, and it now says that it is helping developing countries to find alternatives.[245]

Despite such protestations, however, there is little evidence that the Bank is actually doing this on the ground. Recent Bank policy has reiterated the opinion that user fees are a necessary reform in Africa.[246] In Uganda the government abolished user fees for health services, despite World Bank advice that the policy would have only a minimal impact on attendance at hospitals and clinics. Subsequent events showed that the Ugandan government was well advised to ignore the Bank in this way.[247]

Even with the promises made in 2005 at Gleneagles, by 2010 rich countries will only be giving 0.36 per cent of their income in aid — the same proportion as in 1987.

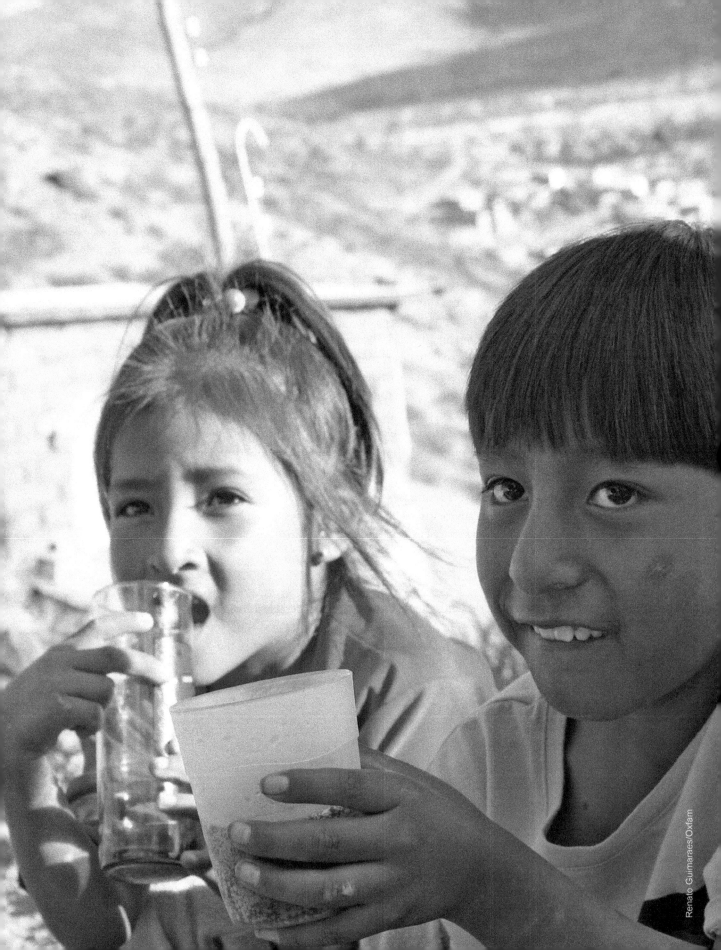

Conclusion

Imagine a world in which for the first time in history, every child is in school. Every woman can give birth with the best possible chance that neither she nor her baby will die. Everyone can drink water without risking their life. Millions of new health workers and teachers are saving lives and shaping minds.

With the Millennium Development Goals, the world's governments have created a platform, and a test of their commitment to end world poverty. We know how to do it: political leadership, government action, and public services, supported by long-term flexible aid from rich countries and the cancellation of debt. We know that the market alone cannot do it, that civil society is picking up some of the pieces, but that governments must act. There is no short cut, and no other way.

To get there, poor country governments must fulfil their responsibilities, their citizens must pressure them to do so, and rich countries must support and not undermine them. In the words of Nelson Mandela:[248]

> 'Poverty is not natural. It is man-made and it can be overcome and eradicated by the actions of human beings. And overcoming poverty is not a gesture of charity. It is an act of justice. It is the protection of a fundamental human right; the right to dignity and a decent life. While poverty persists, there is no freedom.'

opposite page
Children from the Villa Potosi neighbourhood in Cochabamba, Bolivia. The local community have organised themselves to build up the water and sanitation structure, in the hope that they will be able to connect it to the system that serves the rest of the city.

Notes

1   See UN Department of Economic and Social Affairs, The Convention on the Elimination of All Forms of Discrimination against Women (CEDAW); United Nations, Convention on the Rights of the Child (CRC); and UN Economic and Social Council, General Comment No.15: The right to water (Articles 11 and 12 of the International Covenant on Economic, Social and Cultural Rights). The right to clean drinking water was included in the UN's Universal Declaration of Human Rights (1958) and in the CRC in 1989 (Article 24).

2   Calculated from various studies estimating global costs per sector. Education: $10 billion in extra external aid needed per year to achieve Universal Primary Education (e.g. see Doney and Wroe, 2006).
Basic health care: the Macroeconomics and Health Commission estimated an extra $21 billion in external aid needed per year (WHO 2001). Toubkiss estimates from various studies that achieving the water and sanitation MDGs needs $15-20 billion in extra investments per year (Toubkiss 2006, p.7).

3   Canned Food Industry Association, September 2004. www.cannedfood.org (last checked August 2006).

4   The gender parity target has been missed in 94 out of 149 countries where data are available (UNESCO 2006).

5   E. Gomez Gomez 2002.

6   UNDP, Human Development Report 2005.

7   World Health Organization (a).

8   Ibid.

9   Malkin 2006.

10   World Health Organization (a).

11   Malkin 2006.

12   Watkins 2006.

13   Ibid.

14   WaterAid 2005a.

15   World Health Organization (b).

16   UNAIDS/WHO 2005.

17   UN Department of Economic and Social Affairs 2005b.

18   UNAIDS 2004, p.40.

19   UNICEF (a).

20   UN Department of Economic and Social Affairs 2005a.

21   Except for Eastern Asia and European countries of the CIS, which started out with 90 per cent enrolment rates or higher. United Nations 2005.

22   UNESCO 2005b.

23 The Universal Declaration of Human Rights states: 'Everyone has the right to education. Education shall be free, at least in the elementary and fundamental stages' (Article 26). In addition, the World Declaration of Education for All, the Convention on the Rights of the Child, and the Convention on Discrimination Against Women all recognise the central importance of 'education for all'.

24 Education For All (EFA) and the Jomtien Declaration provide a new global vision for basic education and a global commitment to achieving it (UNESCO (b)). The Dakar Framework for Action, agreed in 2000, outlines new ways of working and processes for governments and the international community to move towards achieving this global commitment (UNESCO (a)). The MDGs provide quantifiable goals and targets by which to measure progress and success, and a recognition that achieving Education For All requires a partnership of developing country governments and international donors.

25 The Fast Track Initiative was set up so that no country seriously committed to EFA would be thwarted by a lack of funding (World Bank (a)).

26 UNESCO (2005) Education for All Global Monitoring Report 2006. UNESCO: Paris, p.319.

27 UNDP 2005c.

28 Davey 2000.

29 Two country scores are created. The first is the essential services rank, determined by performance in four social outcome indicators: child survival (under-five mortality rate per 1,000 population, 2003); schooling (net primary enrolment rate, 2002–03); access to water (percentage of the population with access to improved drinking water, 2002); and access to sanitation (percentage of population with sanitation, 2002). The second is the income rank: countries are ranked according to income per capita (GNI in purchasing power parity, World Bank World Development Indicators Database, 2004).
    The performance of countries in providing essential services can then be compared with their income. The index is an indicative tool for comparison only and, while the greatest care has been taken to use cross-country data from reliable sources, scores are highly sensitive to data weaknesses and have no explanatory power. For sources of data, see:
    www.childinfo.org/areas/childmortality/u5data.php (UNICEF);
    http://hdr.undp.org/statistics/data/indicators.cfm?x=117&y=1&z=1 (UNDP);
    www.childinfo.org/areas/water/countrydata.php (UNICEF);
    www.childinfo.org/areas/sanitation/countrydata.php (UNICEF) (last accessed August 2006).

30 This section draws heavily on Colclough 1997 and Sen 1999.

31 Public Services International Research Unit 2003.

32 Ibid.

33 UNDP, Human Development Report 2005, p.58.

34 Ibid.

35 Selected by region for their rapid and above-average achievements in health and education. See Mehrotra and Jolly (eds) 1997, chapter 2 for more detail about how countries were selected.

36 Dates of 'breakthrough' periods in under-five mortality reduction ranged from the 1940s to the 1990s. See Mehrotra and Jolly (eds.) 1997, p.66 for details.

37   Case study countries were notable for all having started with enrolment rates higher than regional averages. By the 1980s all case study countries had achieved near 100 per cent net primary enrolment rates for both girls and boys and higher than average secondary enrolments for both girls and boys. See Mehrotra and Jolly (eds.) 1997, p.88 for details.

38   World Development Report 2004, p.59.

39   Ibid.

40   Melrose 1985 and Garfield and Williams 1989.

41   See for example, Mehrotra and Jolly (eds.) 1997. From a wide sample of developing countries, Mehrotra and Jolly selected countries that had consistently higher health and education outcome indicators than the respective regional average for most sectors. Outcome indicators (disaggregated by gender) included infant mortality rate, maternal mortality rate, life expectancy at birth, adult literacy, and primary school enrolments. Hence countries may not have been high achievers in the absolute sense, but were high-performing for their region.

42   Mehrotra 2004.

43   In South Korea, health care was provided primarily through private health insurance, with the state funding free medical assistance for the poor.

44   Mehrotra and Jolly (eds.) 1997, p.432. In Kerala, for example, 60 per cent of schools are private for-profit enterprises. 'Kerala regulates and monitors these private schools by paying the salaries of all teachers, whether private or public, and all private schools are regulated, inspected, and monitored by the state to ensure quality and conformity to standards.'

45   See Rannan-Eliya and Somanathan 2005. The study included national insurance health systems in Japan, Korea, Taiwan, Thailand, and Mongolia; non-universal, tax-funded health systems in Bangladesh, Indonesia, India, and Nepal; 'transition' health systems in China and Viet Nam; and universal, tax-funded systems in Sri Lanka, Malaysia, and Hong Kong.

46   Falling mortality in Sri Lanka, Kerala, and Zimbabwe seems to have been achieved initially in spite of low water and sanitation coverage. See Mehrotra and Jolly (eds.) 1997, p.81.

47   Herz and Sperling 2004, p.85.

48   Ibid., p.87.

49   See Bennell 2004, p.18.

50   Ndong-Jatta, A.T. (2002) 'Providing Quality Basic Education for All: A New Focus', presentation by Gambian Secretary of Education, 11 June 2002. Quoted by Herz and Sperling, 2004, p.61.

51   Health and education spending ranged from 5–8 per cent of GDP and was higher per capita in all countries, well above their respective regional averages.

52   Net primary enrolment rate. Herz and Sperling 2004, p.75, p.87.

53   Education's share of the national budget rose from 22 per cent to 31 per cent in 1999, cutting the defence budget in the process. Herz and Sperling 2004, p.87.

54   User fees were abolished towards the end of 2000/01. Outpatient attendance increased by 84 per cent between 2000/01 and 2002/03, and doubled in some districts. Yates et al. 2006, p.347.

55   Deininger and Mpuga 2004.

56   International AIDS Society 2005.

57   This was achieved because Brazil was able to manufacture its own generic ARVs to keep the cost of the drugs down. However, this only applied to first-line drugs. Second-line drugs, which are needed to counter resistance to first-line drugs after prolonged treatment, are seriously threatened by the high cost of branded ARVs.

58   See Chequer 2005.

59   See Maltz 2005, pp.29-36.

60   Department of Drinking Water Supply, Ministry of Rural Development, Government of India, 2004, Total Sanitation Campaign. http://ddws.nic.in/tsc-nic/html/index.htm.

61   See Santiago 2005.

62   Narayan et al. 2000.

63   Adult female literacy in Yemen was 31 per cent in 2003. WHO, http://www.emro.who.int/emrinfo/index.asp?Ctry=yem (last checked by the author April 2006).

64   Only 28 per cent of deliveries were attended by trained personnel in 2003, according to WHO. http://www.emro.who.int/emrinfo/index.asp?Ctry=yem (last checked by the author April 2006).

65   The prevalence of child malnutrition (percentage of children under five) was 38.1 per cent in 1995. The under-five infant mortality rate was 114 per 1,000 live births in 2002 (WHO). http://www.emro.who.int/cbi/PDF/MDG/Yemen/MDG%20Yemen%20Country%20Profile.htm (last checked by the author April 2006).

66   Bagash 2003.

67   Personal communication with Oxfam GB staff in 2005, anonymity requested.

68   www.jctr.org.zm/bnb/may06.html.

69   USAID 2003, p.11.

70   Refers to doctors, nurses, midwives, and health support staff (WHO 2006).

71   Based on Oxfam calculations.

72   The High Level Forum on Health Millennium Development Goals concluded that the biggest bottleneck in the fight against AIDS is the critical lack of health personnel (cited in UNAIDS 2005).

73   Education For All Fast Track Initiative indicative benchmark of one trained teacher for every 40 primary school-age children. See World Bank 2004.

74   Based on the Joint Learning Initiative study (2004) minimum of 2.5 health workers per 1,000 population, or 400 people for each health worker.

75   Liberia, Uganda, Central African Republic, Mali, Chad, Eritrea, Ethiopia, Rwanda, Somalia, and the Gambia. Oxfam calculations 2006. Based on data from Joint Learning Initiative 2004.

76   Joint Learning Initiative 2004.

77   Anthony Harries, Malawi Ministry of Health, Technical Adviser HIV Care and Support. Quoted in Nolen 2005.

78   Nolen 2005.

79   Dovlo and Nyonator 1999.

80   Joint Learning Initiative 2004, p.28.

81   The willingness of households to pay for services is differentiated on the basis of income, gender, and other factors. Where women and girls have a low status in society, making households pay often means that women and girls are much less likely to access services. See de Vogli and Birbeck 2005.

82   See Gilson 1997.

83   Survey (2005) by Bentaoet-Kattan, for UNESCO 2006.

84   In low-income countries as much as 70 per cent of health spending consists of private, out-of-pocket payments to private providers (World Bank 2005, p.90). For example, in Nigeria, Cambodia, and India private health spending is at least 70 per cent of total national health spending (see Vyas and Palmer 2005).

85   Maternal deaths in the Zaria region of Nigeria rose by 56 per cent, while there was a decline of 46 per cent in the number of deliveries in the main hospital. Nanda 2002, p.129.

86   Nair, Kirbat, and Sexton 2004.

87   In Philips et al. 2004.

88   Ibid.

89   Médecins Sans Frontières 2004.

90   Belli et al. 2002.

91   Personal communication with author, April 2006.

92   See Koblinsky 2003, p.2.

93   Collingnon and Vezina 2000, in Moran and Batley 2004.

94   McIntosh 2003, p.47.

95   Both stats in Vyas and Palmer 2005.

96   Rose and Akyeampong 2005.

97   Calaguas 2005.

98   DFID (unpublished paper).

99   The share of education in national income (GNP) increased between 1998 and 2002 in about two-thirds of countries for which there are data (UNESCO 2006). Between 1990 and 2002, education spending rose from an average of 12 per cent to 14 per cent of government spending; this trend was most pronounced in sub-Saharan Africa, South Asia, Europe, and Central Asia (World Bank 2005).

100   Government education spending in North America and Western Europe rarely reaches 15 per cent of the national budget; more than half of the countries in sub-Saharan Africa with data available surpass this level. UNESCO 2006.

101   Studies estimate that putting every child in the world in a good quality primary school would cost between $7 billion and $17 billion a year (Delamonica, Mehrotra, and Vandemoortele 2001; UNESCO 2002; Oxfam International 2001; Devarajan, Miller, and Swanson 2002; Bruns, Mingat, and Rakotomalala 2003; and Sperling 2003 — all cited in UNDP 2005c). The Global Campaign for Education (2005) states that aid to basic education should reach at least $10 billion by 2010, or about 20 per cent of the total $48 billion increase promised at the G8 in Gleneagles in 2005.

102 For example, between 1990 and 2002 government spending on healthin low-income countriesincreased from 5 per cent to 7 per cent. World Bank 2005b, p.90.

103 The Commission on Macroeconomics and Health found that a set of essential health interventions costs around $34 per person per year as an absolute minimum. The Commission estimates that least developed countries will be able to mobilise around $15 per person per year by 2007, leaving a gap of $19 per person per year. See WHO 2001, p.11.

104 Figures refer to all investments, aid, taxes, and private investments. Global funding estimates vary from $9–$30 billion per year depending on the source of the estimate. However, if the estimates are analysed on comparable parameters, there is a much smaller range of around $10 billion per year to supply low-cost water and sanitation services to people not currently supplied, and a further $15–$20 billion to maintain current services and improve service quality. If the collection and treatment of household wastewater and the maintenance of integrated water management is included, the estimate increases to up to $80 billion. Toubkiss 2006, p.7.

105 Essential health interventions are estimated to cost around 10 per cent of GNP in least developed countries, with a tax take estimated at 14 per cent of GNP. WHO 2001, p.57.

106 Of the 36 countries in the world that spend more on their military than on health or education and for which data are available, these ten have the worst score in the Human Development Index. Data from UNDP 2005a.

107 Hospitals and universities are a necessary part of essential services — universities train doctors and nurses, and urban and district hospitals are often used by poor people too. The problem comes when too much public money is spent on services used by a minority. For example, a single specialised, urban-based referral hospital can take up 20 per cent of the entire government budget, whereas the patterns of disease in many developing countries indicate a need to prioritise spending on rural health centres and district hospitals for the health-care needs of the majority.

108 Only six out of 21 countries for which data were available (Sri Lanka, Nicaragua, Colombia, Costa Rica, Honduras, Argentina) spent as much or more on health services for the poorest fifth of the population as they did on services for the richest fifth. Only four countries out of 35 (Colombia, Jamaica, Romania, Costa Rica) for which data were available spent as much or more on education services for the poorest fifth of the population as on services for the richest fifth. Based on total health and total education spending, Filmer 2003 in World Bank 2004a, p.39.

109 World Development Report 2006. Washington, DC: World Bank.

110 Paxson and Schady 2005.

111 World Bank, World Development Report 2006.

112 WaterAid Nepal 2002/2004 and WaterAid 2006.

113 UNDP 2005a.

114 UNDP 2005a.

115 UNDP 2005a.

116 The interviewee requested anonymity.

117 For instance, the World Bank is currently investigating mis-procurement in 43 contracts linked to seven of its projects in Cambodia, and has found types of corruption including solicitation and acceptance of bribes, price fixing, and colluding to manipulate tenders and inflate bid prices.
See http://web.worldbank.org (last checked by the author July 2006).

118 Elshorst and O'Leary 2005.

119 World Development Report 2004.

120 Transparency International, *Global Corruption Report 2006*.

121 Meier and Griffin 2005.

122 *Global Corruption Report*.

123 Kessler and Alexander 2003.

124 Barrientos 2000.

125 Patient choice is unlikely to explain the high rate of Caesareans. At a private clinic where 70 per cent of women have Caesarean sections, only 18 per cent requested them. Murray 2000.

126 Hao et al. 1997, cited in Mehrotra and Delamonica 2005, p.155.

127 Public Services International Research Unit (PSIRU) 2002.

128 Kruse and Ramos 2003. Privatisation of the municipal water board SEMAPA was a condition of a 1996 loan and of HIPC debt relief in 1997.

129 The consortium Aguas del Tunari (AdT) was led by International Water Limited, a company jointly owned by the US multinational Bechtel and the Italian energy company Edison.

130 Cited in various sources, including Palast in the *Guardian* (2000).
www.guardian.co.uk/Archive/Article/0,4273,4010929,00.html (last checked by the author July 2006).

131 Reports of price hikes vary from 35 per cent (e.g. Palast 2000) to 300 per cent (Kruse and Ramos 2003). Braun (2004) states that hikes in water prices averaged 51 per cent.

132 Alexander 2005, p.19.

133 There are numerous reports on the riots, including Kruse and Ramos 2003.

134 In February 2002, AdT filed a case with the World Bank's International Centre for the Settlement of Investment Disputes (ICSID) based on a bilateral investment treaty between Bolivia and the Netherlands, where Bechtel's subsidiary, International Water Co., had established a presence. AdT and Bechtel sought $25m in damages for breach of their 40-year, multi-million-dollar contract. See Alexander (2005, p.19).

135 International Water and Sanitation Centre 2006.

136 Lethbridge 2002, p.19.

137 Estache and Rossi 2002, p.139.

138 Estache, Perelman, and Trujillo 2005, p.21. A recent study of the distributional impact of privatisation found that most privatisation programmes worsened the distribution of assets and incomes, at least in the short run. Birdsall and Nellis 2002.

139 Estache 2004, p.10.

140 Bayliss 2001.

141 Hornblow, A., 'New Zealand's health reforms: a clash of cultures', *British Medical Journal*, http://bmj.bmjjournals.com/cgi/content/full/314/7098/1892.

142 Schick1998.

143 IMF Public Private Partnerships, 12 March 2004.

144 Mehrotra and Delamonica 2005, p.165.

145 This critique draws heavily on Watt, P. 'Comment on draft 2004 World Development Report', ActionAid, May 2003.

146 See p.13 and p.107 of the 2004 World Development Report.

147 Wood 2005a. Conditions come in a range of guises, from the strongest (prior actions) to the weakest (benchmarks). All have an influence on country policy.

148 EURODAD 2006, p.3.

149 HIPC is now the Multilateral Debt Relief Initiative.

150 '…more than half the countries which have reached Decision Point will be (or have been) required to implement reforms concerning public-private partnership, commercialisation or outright privatisation of SOEs to meet Completion Point.' Jubilee Debt Campaign (forthcoming).

151 Mehrotra and Delamonica 2005, p.165.

152 A target contained in the Private Sector Development Strategy 2002. Mehrotra and Delamonica 2005, p.165.

153 Ibid., p.166.

154 Ibid.

155 'When private firms lend to or invest in a water project in a borrowing country, the Bank's guarantee promises the private firms compensation for certain losses if, under specified conditions, the borrower does not meet its obligations.' Kessler 2004, p.8.

156 Cliff Stone, the British chief executive of City Water, 'accepted that the project was well behind schedule and that no new pipes had been installed, but claimed water quality and quantity had improved and that 10,000 new customers had been signed up in the last two months.' Vidal 2005.

157 The initial privatisation proposal failed to attract any bidders and Tanzania was granted a waiver on the HIPC trigger and provided with debt relief anyway. The World Bank's push to privatise DAWASA continued through a $143 million scheme which eventually resulted in the awarding of a contract to City Water — a partnership made up of Biwater, Gauff (a German engineering company), and the Tanzanian company Superdall — to provide services in Dar es Salaam and the surrounding region. A case was filed by City Water against the Tanzanian government for alleged breach of contract. Greenhill and Weklya 2004; Vidal 2005, http://www.guardian.co.uk/hearafrica05/story/0,15756,1491600,00.html (last checked by the author April 2006).

158 Birdsall and Nellis 2002.

159 Hall and de la Motte 2005.

160 Greenhill and Weklya 2004.

161 Vidal 2005. Adam Smith International is a sister organisation to UK free market thinktank the Adam Smith Institute.

162   The UK Department for International Development's policy on conditionality explicitly states that privatisation should not be pushed using conditions on aid (see DFID 2005b). The EC in a 2003 paper concluded that privatisation of utilities and other state-owned enterprises had been pushed 'without looking at all the options' and that the Commission had supported this by linking its aid to World Bank and IMF programmes where privatisation had been a condition (see Commission of the European Communities 2003). The new Norwegian government has stated that 'Norwegian aid should not go to programmes that contain requirements for liberalisation and privatisation' (see Norwegian Labour Party 2006).

163   Sondorp 2004.

164   Vyas and Palmer 2005.

165   Rose and Akyeampong 2005; and BRAC 2005.

166   Palmer and Mills (2006).

167   Ibid.

168   Ibid.

169   Education International (2005).

170   BBC News (2005) 'UK Crippling Africa Healthcare', http://news.bbc.co.uk/1/hi/health/4582283.stm (last checked by the author March 2006).

171   Joint Learning Initiative 2004.

172   Mehrotra 2004b.

173   World Bank 2005b.

174   Dugger, C. 'U.S. plan to lure nurses may hurt poor nations', *New York Times*, 24 May 2006.

175   OECD/DAC 2005a.

176   Oxfam International 2006.

177   The data here represent aid to basic education, basic health care, reproductive health, and water supply and sanitation for 2004. They are commitment data, not disbursement data. The figures are measured as a proportion of total aid, not sector-allocable aid, which disadvantages donors such as DFID, which now funnel much aid to basic social services through budget support. They may also overestimate aid to basic services, as they take a broader measure of water supply and sanitation than that defined for essential services by Oxfam. OECD/DAC database, accessed on 2 March 2006. http://www.oecd.org.

178   Bokhari, Gottret, and Gai (2005) 'Government Health Expenditures, Donor Funding and Health Outcomes' cited in World Bank 2006, p.61. The study suggests that aid volatility imposes a significant constraint on the ability of governments to spend health money effectively.

179   In 2001/02 some 53 per cent of aid for water and sanitation needs went to just ten countries — only four of which were low-income. On the whole, countries that were favoured with relatively high amounts of aid for water and sanitation received $447 per un-served person, while the neediest low-income countries received just $16 per un-served person. Tearfund 2004.

180   It is projected that 1.8 million people will receive antiretroviral treatment over the next five years with Global Fund resources. More than 1 million orphans will be supported through medical services, education, and community care (rounds one to three of funding). Global Fund website (last checked by the author 5 May 2006). www.theglobalfund.org/en/about/aids/default.asp.

181   Ibid.

182   Global Fund website,
      http://www.theglobalfund.org/en/files/about/replenishment/replenishment_pledges_2006_2007.pdf.

183   'We in fact in the Bank now are quite embarrassed with a number of countries that are ready to go on
      Education for All, do not have the money, but have very good plans that are well-integrated and
      well-supported, and they say to us, "Well, now, we have done what you have asked us to do —
      where is the money?".' World Bank 2004 Spring Meetings, press conference with James D. Wolfensohn.
      Washington, DC, 22 April 2004. http://web.worldbank.org.

184   Progress report prepared for the EFA-FTI partnership meeting, December 2005. Washington, DC:
      FTI Secretariat. www.fasttrackinitiative.org.

185   See, for example, Oxfam International press release, 'Zambia uses G8 debt cancellation to make health care
      free for the poor', 31 March 2006 and http://allafrica.com/stories/200603310782.html.

186   ActionAid International 2005, p.21.

187   Known as Dutch disease because the Netherlands experienced a decrease in its competitiveness following
      the discovery and subsequent export of natural gas reserves in the 1960s.

188   Foster and Killick 2006.

189   OECD/DAC 2005b.

190   World Bank 2006, p.63.

191   Quoted in Stillman and Bennett 2005.

192   Quoted in WaterAid 2005b.

193   World Bank 2005b, p.93.

194   The single most expensive item in an education system is the salary bill, which accounted for more than
      70 per cent of education costs in most of 47 low-income countries studied by Bruns et al. in 2003.

195   World Bank 2006, p.60.

196   Personal communication with report author, Richard Jolly, Institute of Development Studies,
      University of Sussex.

197   Personal communication with Oxfam GB staff.

198   'La Realidad de la Ayuda 2004/5', Intermon Oxfam, Madrid.

199   OECD/DAC database, last searched by author August 2006.

200   Stillman and Bennett 2005.

201   'The Global Fund is taking away human resources from diseases such as malaria to VCT [voluntary testing
      and counselling for HIV/AIDS], where there are funds.' Donor representative quoted in Stillman and
      Bennett 2005.

202   Oxfam 2004.

203   Social Watch 2005.

204   Reis and Moore 2005.

205   Ibid.

206 *Equals* Issue 2, 2003, p.5. Newsletter for Beyond Access: Gender, Education and Development.
     August 2003, London: Institute of Education.

207 World Bank 2005a, p.22.

208 Burns et al 2005.

209 Adams 2001, p.2.

210 Herz and Sperling 2004.

211 Pitanguy 1994.

212 Chisholm and McKinney 2003, pp.8-9.

213 Assembly figures from UN statistics:
     http://unstats.un.org/unsd/demographic/products/indwm/ww2005/tab6.htm (last accessed 4 April 2006).

214 Joshi and Fawcett 2005.

215 In 1994 the Presidential Lead Programme introduced free health care for pregnant women and children
     under six. A national evaluation in 1995 showed 20–60 per cent increases in total health utilisation at
     13 sites (Gilson 2003), and pregnant women started to attend antenatal care facilities at an earlier stage
     (McCoy 1996, in McIntyre et al. 2005). In 1996 the Minister of Health announced free primary health care.
     The impact of this policy has never been comprehensively analysed, but a panel household survey in one
     rural province showed 'quite large increases in the use of public sector primary care facilities after this
     policy — though the increase was below average for the poorest group' (personal communication from
     Dr. Jane Goudge, Centre for Health Policy, to McIntyre et al. 2005).

216 This investment would cover the current revenue from fees and the increased value of user fees that would
     result when utilisation rates increase. See Save the Children 2005.

217 Community-based health insurance schemes provide basic medical cover that is paid for by small
     pre-payments from community members. The difference is that user fees are charged at the point of
     delivery, whereas insurance schemes pool up-front contributions.

218 In common with other community-based health financing mechanisms, revenue raised from member fees
     in Oxfam's own scheme covers 80 per cent of the cost of drugs, but only around 30 per cent of the total cost of
     providing the service. For this reason the scheme operates with considerable subsidy from Oxfam and other
     donors and is intended as a stopgap until such time as the state can take over the operating costs.

219 For example, Uganda experimented with community-based health insurance schemes from 1995 to 2002.
     A series of reviews concluded that such schemes did not cover their costs, failed to reach the poorer members
     of the communities they served, and were mildly regressive in that they used public money to subsidise access
     to services by the somewhat better-off. Given these concerns, the Ministry of Health decided not to scale up
     insurance schemes, but chose instead to abolish user fees in public health clinics. Yates et al 2006, pp.345-6.

220 Calaguas 2005.

221 Miranda 2005 in Balanyá et al 2005 (eds.).

222 Hallack, J. and M. Poisson (2005) 'Ethics and corruption in education', *Journal of Education for
     International Development*. http://www.equip123.net/JEID/articles/1/1-3.pdf.

223 *Global Corruption Report*, p.65.

224   Transparency International 2006, p.120.

225   Personal communication with the author from the head of the Law Society in Malawi.

226   For example, see Kane 2004, p.105.

227   See SIDA 2005.

228   See WaterAid 2005b.

229   Martin 1997.

230   Sumra 2004.

231   Public Services International Research Unit 2005.

232   Mugisha, Berg, and Muhairwe (forthcoming) cited in Calaguas 2005.

233   Transparency International 2006.

234   UNESCO 2005b, p.184.

235   See USAID 2003, p.26.

236   WaterAid 2005b.

237   Birdsall, Levine, and Ibrahim 2005.

238   For example, central government revenues account for around one-third of GDP in Europe, whereas total tax take, including trade and indirect taxes, in poorer regions (South Asia, sub-Saharan Africa, Middle-East/North Africa, etc.) is generally around 15 per cent of GDP. Cobham 2005, pp.6-8.

239   Baunsguaard, T. and M. Keen, 'Tax Revenue or Trade Liberalisation', IMF working paper, June 2005.

240   A breakdown of projects in the health sector in Uganda between 1997-98 and 2002-03 shows that they were highly inefficient: 68 per cent went on inputs that were not included in the Health Sector Strategy, such as technical assistance, capacity building, and project overheads. Presentation to Oxfam GB by Rob Yates, advisor to Ministry of Health, Uganda.

241   Based on a joint survey for OECD/DAC over five years of budget support in Burkina Faso, Malawi, Mozambique, Nicaragua, Rwanda, Uganda, and Viet Nam. University of Birmingham (forthcoming). A summary of the research can be found at: www.oecd.org/dataoecd/16/31/36644712.pdf (last checked by author May 2006). Other studies noting significant gains from budget support under the right political conditions include High Level Forum on Health (2003) and EQUINET (2004).

242   Lawson et al. 2005.

243   Merlin 2005, pp.32-33.

244   DFID 2004, pp.3-7.

245   'The World Bank does not support user fees for primary education and basic health services for poor people. Access to these basic services is vital to improving the welfare of the poor in developing countries. Experience shows that, particularly in relation to education, user fees restrict the ability of poor people to send their children to school. The Bank also supports provision of free basic health services and helps countries find alternative means to finance these activities.' World Bank 2003.

246   'Publicly subsidised care for all is not an affordable option for African governments.' World Bank 2004.

247 Earlier World Bank modelling had suggested that the policy change would result in a 2.3 per cent increase in utilisation. In fact, removing user fees in health resulted in a roughly 80 per cent increase in use. Personal communication from Yates (2004) to the author.

248 Nelson Mandela (2005), speech for Make Poverty History Campaign. http://news.bbc.co.uk/1/hi/uk_politics/4232603.stm.

References

ActionAid International (2005) 'Contradicting Commitments: How the Achievement of Education for All is Being Undermined by the International Monetary Fund', http://www.actionaid.org/wps/content/documents/contradicting_1892005_104812.pdf (last checked by the author April 2006).

ActionAid International and Global Campaign for Education (2005) 'Educate to End Poverty — Why the UN Must Make Girls' Education its Number One Priority at the Millennium + 5 Summit', http://www.actionaidusa.org/pdf/educatetoendpovertypaper2.pdf (last checked by the author April 2006).

Adams, J. (2001) 'Women and social security: how far are we?' IDASA Budget Brief No. 75.

Alexander, N. (2005) 'The Roles Of The IMF, The World Bank, And The WTO In Liberalization And Privatisation Of The Water Services Sector', Citizens Network On Essential Services, Maryland, USA.

Barrientos, A.(2000) 'Getting better after neo-liberalism — shifts and challenges of health policy in Chile', *Healthcare Reform and Poverty in Latin America*, 94-11.

Bagash, T. (2003) 'Project Context and Policy Environment', paper for Oxfam GB in Yemen, October 2003.

Balanyá, B. et al. (eds.) (2005) *Reclaiming Public Water*, Amsterdam: Transnational Institute and Corporate Europe Observatory, January 2005.

Bangladesh Rural Advancement Committee (BRAC) Annual Report 2005, Dhaka, Bangladesh.

Bayliss, K. (2001) 'Water Privatisation In Africa, Lessons From Three Case Studies,' Public Services International Research Unit (PSIRU).

BBC News (2005) 'UK crippling Africa healthcare', http://news.bbc.co.uk/1/hi/health/4582283.stm (last checked by the author March 2006).

Belli, P., Shahriari, H. and Curtio Medical Group (2002) 'Qualitative Study on Informal Payments for Health Services in Georgia', World Bank Health, Nutrition and Population (HNP) Discussion Paper 2002.

Bennell, P. (2004) 'Teacher Motivation and Incentives in Sub-Saharan Africa and Asia', Brighton: Knowledge for Skills and Development.

Birdsall, N., Levine, R., and A. Ibrahim (2005) *Toward Universal Primary Education: Investments, Incentives and Institutions*, New York: Millennium Project Task Force on Education and Gender Equality, p.137.

Birdsall, N. and J. Nellis (2002) 'Winners and Losers: Assessing the Distributional Impact of Privatization', Center for Global Development, Working Paper No. 6.

Braun, W. (2004) 'Campesinos vs oil industry', www.zmag.org, December.

Bruns, B., Mingat, A., and R. Rakoomalala (2003), 'Achieving UPE by 2015: A chance for every child', World Bank 2003.

Burnham, G. M., Pariyo, G., Galiwango, E., and F. Wabwire-Mangen (2004) 'Discontinuation of cost sharing in Uganda' in *Bulletin of the World Health Organization*, March 2004, vol. 82 (3).

Burns, J., Keswell, M., and M. Leibbrandt (2005) 'Social assistance, gender and the aged in South Africa' in *Feminist Economics* 11 (2).

Calaguas, B. (2005) 'Improving Water and Sanitation', background paper by WaterAid for Oxfam GB.

Center for Global Development (2004) 'Millions Saved: Proven Successes in Global Health,' CGD Brief Vol. 3(3), October 2004, Washington, DC: Center for Global Health.

Chequer, P. (2005) 'Access to Treatment and Prevention: Brazil and Beyond,' presentation at International AIDS Society Third Conference on HIV Pathogenesis and Treatment. www.ias-2005.org/planner/Presentations/ppt/3333.

Chisholm, L. and C. McKinney (2003) 'Reforms, Innovations and Approaches Used to Work with Teachers to Use Them as Change Agents and Facilitators of Gender Equality in Different Countries: Strengths and Limitations', UNESCO education portal accessed on 4 April 2006. http://portal.unesco.org.

Cobham, A. (2005) 'Taxation Policy and Development', OCGG Economy Analysis no. 2, Oxford: Oxford Council on Good Governance.

Colclough, C. (1997) *Marketising Education and Health in Developing Countries: Miracle or Mirage*, Oxford: Clarendon Press.

Commission Of The European Communities (2003) 'The Reform Of State-Owned Enterprises In Developing Countries With A Focus On Public Utilities: The Need To Assess All The Options', Communication From The Commission To The Council And European Parliament, Brussels, June 2003.

Davey, S. (2000) *Health: A Key to Prosperity. Success Stories in Developing Countries*, Geneva: WHO, CDS.

Delannoy, F. and G. Sedlacek (2000) *Brazil: Teachers' Development and Incentives: A Strategic Framework*. World Bank Report 20408-BR. Washington, D.C.: World Bank.

Deininger, K. and P. Mpuga (2004) 'Economic and Welfare Effects of the Abolition of Health User Fees: Evidence from Uganda', World Bank Policy Research Working Paper 3276, April 2004.

De Vogli, R. and G.L. Birbeck (2005) 'Potential impact of adjustment policies on vulnerability of women and children to HIV/AIDS in sub-Saharan Africa', *Journal of Health and Population Nutrition*, 23(2):105–120.

DFID (2004) 'Improving Health in Malawi: Programme Memorandum November 2004', London: Department For International Development.

DFID (2005a) 'Non-State Providers of Basic Services — A DFID-Funded, Multi-Country Study', presentation at water network meeting, London, April 2005.

DFID (2005b) 'Partnerships For Poverty Reduction: Rethinking Conditionality'. http://www.dfid.gov.uk/pubs/files/conditionality.pdf (last checked by the author April 2006).

Doney, M. and M. Wroe (2006) 'Keeping our promises: delivering education for all', London: HM Treasury and DFID.

Dovlo, D. and F. Nyonator (1999) 'Migration of graduates of the University of Ghana Medical School: a preliminary rapid appraisal', *Human Resources for Health Development Journal*, 1:42-54.

Education International (2005), 'Brain Drain: Rich Country Seeks Poor Teachers', Brussels: Education International.

Elshorst, H. and D. O'Leary (2005) 'Corruption in the Water Sector: Opportunities for Addressing a Pervasive Problem', Transparency International.
http://www.siwi.org/downloads/WWW-Symp/Corruption_in_the_water_sector_Elshorst.pdf.

EQUINET (2004) 'Ensuring universal treatment access through sustainable public health systems', EQUINET discussion document, February 2004.

Ekman, B. (2004) 'Community-based health insurance in low-income countries: a systematic review of the evidence', *Health Policy and Planning*, 19(5): 249-270.

Elson, D. and H. Keklik (2002) *'Progress of World's Women 2002: Vol. 2: Gender Equality and the Millennium Development Goals'*, New York: UNIFEM.

Estache, A. (2004) 'PPI Partnerships versus PPI Divorces in Developing Countries', World Bank and Université Libre de Bruxelles, January 2005.

Estache, A., S. Perelman, and M. Trujillo (2005) 'Infrastructure Performance And Reform In Developing And Transition Economies: Evidence Form A Survey Of Productivity Measures', World Bank Policy Research Paper 3514, February 2005.

Estache, A. and M. A. Rossi (2002) 'How different is the efficiency of public and private water companies in Asia?' *World Bank Economic Review*: 16(1); 139-148. IBRD, Washington DC.

EURODAD (2006) 'World Bank and IMF conditionality: a development injustice'.
www.eurodad.org/articles/default.aspx?id=711.

Foster, M. and T. Killick (2006) 'What Would Doubling Aid Mean for Macroeconomic Management in Africa?' Working Paper 264, Overseas Development Institute: London.

Garfield, R. G. and G. Williams (1989) *Health and Revolution: The Nicaraguan Experience*, Oxfam GB: Oxford.

Gilson, L. (2003) 'User Fees: the South African Experience', paper presented at the National Institute of Health, USA, www.fic.nih.gov/dcpp/ppts/gilson1.ppt (last checked by the author April 2006).

Gilson, L. (1997) 'The lessons of user fee experience in Africa', *Health Policy & Planning,* 12(4); 273-85.

Global Campaign for Education (2005) 'UN Millennium Summit Delivers Rhetoric without Commitment', paper presented at the G8 Summit 2005, www.campaignforeducation.org.

Gomez Gomez, E. (2002) *'Gender Equity and Health Policy Reform in Latin America and the Caribbean'*, Washington DC: Pan American Health Organization.

Greenhill, R. and I. Weklya (2004) 'Turning Off The Taps: Donor Conditionality And Water Privatisation In Dar Es Salaam, Tanzania', London, ActionAid International. www.actionaid.org.uk/wps/content/documents/ TurningofftheTAps.pdf (last checked by the author April 2006).

Gutierrez, E. and Y. Musaazi (2003) 'The changing meaning of reforms in Uganda: grappling with privatisation as public water services improve', WaterAid, mimeo.

Hall, L. and R. de la Motte (2005) 'Public resistance to privatisation in water and energy' in *Development in Practice*. Vol 15 No. 3 and 4.

Herz, B. and G.B. Sperling (2004) *What Works in Girls' Education: Evidence and Policies from the Developing World.* New York: Council on Foreign Relations.

High Level Forum on Health (2003) 'Harmonisation and MDGs: a perspective from Tanzania and Uganda'. Conference paper.

Human Development Report (2005) *International Co-operation at a Crossroads: Aid, Trade and Security in an Unequal World*, New York: UNDP.

International AIDS Society (2005) 'Fact Sheet: HIV/AIDS in Brazil and Latin America'. www.ias-2005.org/admin/images/upload/534.pdf (last checked by the author March 2006).

International Monetary Fund (2004) 'Public-Private Partnerships', www.imf.org/external/np/fad/2004/pifp/eng/031204.htm (last checked by the author April 2006).

International Water and Sanitation Centre (2006) 'Bolivia, Cochabamba: public pressure forces Bechtel to drop water case', www.irc.nl/page/27840 (last checked by the author April 2006).

Joint Learning Initiative (2004) *Human Resources for Health: Overcoming the Crisis*. Boston, MA: Harvard University Global Equity Initiative.

Joshi, D. and B. Fawcett (2005) 'The Role of Water in an Unequal Social Order in India' in Coles, A. and T. Wallace (eds) *Gender, Water and Development* (2005), Berg, Oxford.

Jubilee Debt Campaign (forthcoming) 'Tightening the Leash or Loosening the Strings? The status of HIPC conditionality in 2006'.

Kane, E. (2004) 'Girls' education in Africa: what do we know about strategies that work?', Africa Human Development Working Paper Series, Washington DC: World Bank.

Kessler, T. (2004) 'The Pros And Cons Of Private Provision Of Water And Electricity Service: A Handbook For Evaluating Rationales', Citizens' Network on Essential Services. www.servicesforall.org (last checked by the author April 2006).

Kessler, T. and N. Alexander (2003) 'Assessing The Risks In The Private Provision Of Essential Services', Discussion Paper For G-24 Technical Group, Citizens' Network on Essential Services, www.servicesforall.org/html/tools/assessing_risks.shtmlhtml (last checked by the author April 2006).

Koblinsky, M.A. (ed.) (2003) *Reducing Maternal Mortality: Learning from Bolivia, China, Egypt, Honduras, Indonesia, Jamaica and Zimbabwe*, Washington, DC: World Bank.

Kruse, T. and C. Ramos (2003) 'Water privatisation: doubtful benefits, concrete threats' in *Social Watch Report 2003*, Social Watch.

Lafer, G., Moss, H., Kirtner R. and V. Rees (2003) 'Solving the Nursing Shortage: Best and Worst Practices for Recruiting, Retaining and Recouping of Hospital Nurses. A Report Prepared for the United Nurses of America', AFSCME, AFL-CIO, Oregon: Labor Education and Research Center.

Lawson, A., Booth, D., Msuya, M., Wangwe S. and T. Williamson (2005) 'Does General Budget Support Work? Evidence from Tanzania', London: Overseas Development Institute.

Lethbridge, J. (2002) 'Forces and Reactions in Healthcare', PSIRU, December 2002.

Malkin, E. (2006) 'Big-time shift in facing water crisis', *New York Times*, 21 March 2006 www.iht.com/articles/2006/03/20/news/water.php (last checked by the author March 2006).

Maltz, H. (2005) 'Porto Alegre's water: public and for all' in Balanyá et al (eds) (2005) *Reclaiming Public Water*, Transnational Institute.

Martin, B. (1997) 'From clientelism to participation — The story of "participatory budgeting" in Porto Alegre', www.publicworld.org/docs/portoalegre.pdf.

McIntosh, A.C. (2003) *Asian Water Supplies — Reaching the Poor*, Asian Development Bank, Manila and IWA Publishing, London.

McIntyre, D., Gilson. L. and M. Vimbayi (2005) 'Promoting Equitable Health Care Financing in the African Context: Current Challenges and Future Prospects', EQUINET discussion paper no. 27, October 2005.

Médecins Sans Frontières (2004) 'Burundi Deprived of Access to Healthcare', MSF policy paper.

Mehrotra, S. (2004a) 'Improving Child Wellbeing in Developing Countries: What do we know? What can be done?', CHIP report No. 9.

Mehrotra, S. (2004b) 'Reforming Public Spending on Education and Mobilising Resources: Lessons from International Experience', *Economic and Political Weekly*, 28 February 2004.

Mehrotra, S. and E. Delamonica (2005) 'The private sector and privatisation in social services: is the Washington Consensus dead?' *Global Social Policy*, Vol 5 (2).

Mehrotra, S. and P. Buckland (1998) 'Managing Teacher Costs for Access and Quality', UNICEF Staff Working Papers No. EPP-EVL-98-004, New York, NY: UNICEF.

Mehrotra, S. and R. Jolly (eds.) (1997) *Development With A Human Face — Experiences in Social Achievement and Economic Growth,* Clarendon Press: Oxford.

Meier, B. and M. Griffin (2005) *Stealing the Future: Corruption in the Classroom*, Berlin: Transparency International.

Melrose, D. (1985) *Nicaragua: The Threat of a Good Example*, Oxfam GB: Oxford.

Merlin (2005) 'Meeting the Health Millennium Development Goals in Fragile States', proceedings from the Merlin-LSHTM Conference on Fragile States, 23–24 June 2005, London: Merlin.

Mills, A. (1995) 'Improving the Efficiency of Public Sector Health Services in Developing Countries: Bureaucratic versus Market Approaches', HEFP Working Paper.

Moran, D. and R. Batley (2004) 'Literature Review of Non-State Provision of Basic Services', paper commissioned by DFID from Governance Resource Centre, University of Birmingham, UK.

Mugisha, S., Berg S.V. and W.T. Muhairwe (forthcoming) 'Using Internal Incentive Contracts to Improve Water Utility Performance: The Case of Uganda's NWSC', http://bear.cba.ufl.edu/centers/purc/primary/documents/Using_Internal_Incentive_Contracts.pdf.

Murray, S.F. (2000) 'Relations between private health insurance and high rates of Caesarean section in Chile: a quantitative and qualitative study', in *British Medical Journal*, 16 December 2000, 321(7275):1501-5.

Nair, S. and P. Kirbat with Sexton, S. (2004) 'A Decade after Cairo — Women's Health in a Free Market Economy', Cornerhouse Briefing 31, June 2004.

Nanda, P. (2002) 'Gender dimensions of user fees: implications for women's utilisation of health care', *Reproductive Health Matters* 2002; 10 (20) 127-134.

Narayan, D. with Patel, R., Schafft, K., Rademacher A. and S. Koch-Schulte (2000) *Voices of the Poor: Can Anyone Hear Us?* New York, N.Y.: published for the World Bank, Oxford University Press.

National Water and Sewerage Corporation (NWSC) (2005) *Annual Report 2004-2005*, Kampala, Uganda: National Water and Sewerage Corporation.

Nolen, S. (2005) 'Deaths rob Malawi of warriors in its assault against AIDS', *Toronto Globe and Mail*, 21 November 2005.

Norwegian Labour Party (2006) 'The Soria Moria Declaration on International Policy', www.dna.no/index.gan?id=47619&subid=0 (last checked by the author April 2006).

Nyonator, F.K., Awoonor-Williams, J.K., Phillips, J.F., Jones T.C. and R.A. Miller (2005) 'The Ghana Community-based Health Planning and Services Initiative for scaling up service delivery innovation', *Health Policy and Planning*, 2005, 20(1): 25-34.

OECD/DAC (2005a) Paris High-Level Forum on Aid Effectiveness, Paris, France, 2–3 March 2005.

OECD/DAC (2005b) 'Survey on Harmonisation and Alignment: Overview of the Survey Results', www.oecd.org/dataoecd/31/37/33981948.pdf (last checked by the author April 2006).

OECD/DAC Database www.oecd.org/document/31/0,2340,en_2649_34485_33764703_1_1_1_1,00.html (last checked by the author April 2006).

Oxfam (2004) 'Programme Impact Report 2004', Oxford: Oxfam.

Oxfam International (2006) 'The View from the Summit — Gleneagles G8 One Year On', Oxford: Oxfam.

Palmer, N., Mills, A., Wadee, H., Gilson, L., and H. Schneider (2003) 'A New Face For Private Providers In Developing Countries: What Implications For Public Health?', WHO Bulletin, Vol. 81 (4).

Palmer N. and A. Mills (2006) 'Contracting-out health service provision in resource- and information-poor settings' in Jones, A.M. (ed.) *Elgar Companion to Health Economics*, Cheltenham: Edward Elgar, pp.250-258.

Paxson, C.H. and N. Schady (2005), 'Cognitive Development Among Young Children in Ecuador: The Roles of Wealth, Health, and Parenting', Washington, DC: World Bank Policy Research Working Paper Series 3605.

Phillips M., Ooms, G., Hargreaves S. and A. Durrant (2004) 'Burundi: a population deprived of basic health care', *British Journal of General Practice*: 54 (505); 633-48.

Phillips, O. and A. Durrant (2004), 'Burundi: A Population Deprived of Basic Health Care', Geneva: MSF.

Pitanguy, J. (1994) 'Feminist Politics and Reproductive Rights: The Case of Brazil', in Sen G. and R.C. Snow (eds.) *Power and Decision: The Social Control of Reproduction*, Cambridge, MA: Harvard University Press, pp.101-122.

Pritchett, L. (2005) 'The Political Economy of Targeted Safety Nets', Social Protection Discussion Paper Series no. 0501, Washington, DC: World Bank.

Public Services International Research Unit (2002) 'Privatisation Of Basic Services: Concerns About Donor Policies', PSIRU submission to UK International Development Parliamentary Select Committee, November 2002.

Public Services International Research Unit (2003) 'Public Services Work'. www.psiru.org/reports/2003-09-U-PSW.pdf.

Public Services International Research Unit (2005) 'Focus on Public Services'.

Public World (2004) 'Delivering Good Quality Services: Health and Education', report for Oxfam GB.

Rannan-Eliya, R. and A. Somanathan (2005) 'Health Systems, Not Local Projects, Provide the Key to Social Protection for the Poor in Asia', London, DFID Health Systems Resource Centre.

Reis, P. and M. Moore (eds.) 'Elite Perceptions of Poverty and Inequality', Zed, London 2005.

Rose, P.R. and K. Akyeampong (2005) 'The Non-State Sector and Education: Literature Review and Four-Country Study', paper commissioned for Oxfam.

Sachs, J.D. (2001) *Report of the Commission on Macroeconomics and Health,* Geneva: World Health Organization.

Sachs, J.D. (2005) 'Who Beats Corruption?', Project Syndicate: www.project-syndicate.org/print_commentary/sachs106/English (last checked by the author August 2006).

Santiago, C. (2005) 'Public-public partnership: an alternative strategy in water management in Malaysia' in Balanyá, B. et al (eds.) (2005) *Reclaiming Public Water*, Amsterdam: Transnational Institute.

Save the Children (2005) 'Killer Bills: Make Child Poverty History — Abolish User Fees', briefing paper. London: Save the Children.

Schick, A. (1998) 'Why most developing countries should not try New Zealand Reforms', *World Bank Research Observer*, 13(1), February 1998: 723–31.

Sen, A. (1999), *Development as Freedom*, New York, Oxford University Press.

Social Watch (2005) *Roars and Whispers. Gender and Poverty Promises v. Action*. Instituto Del Tercer Mundo, Montevideo, Uruguay.

Sondorp, E. (2004) 'Case Study 1: A Time-Series Analysis of Health Service Delivery in Afghanistan', London: DFID Health Systems Resource Centre.

Stillman, K. and S. Bennett (2005) *Systemwide Effects of the Global Fund: Interim Findings from Three Country Case Studies*, Bethesda, MD: The Partners for Health Reform Plus Project, Abt Associates Inc.

Sumra, S. (2004) 'The Living and Working Conditions of Teachers in Tanzania: A Research Report', Dar es Salaam: HakiElimu.

Swedish International Development Co-operation Agency (SIDA) (2005) www.u4.no/themes/health/healthgoodpracticeex3.cfm (last checked by the author April 2006).

Tearfund (2004) 'Making every drop count: An assessment of donor progress towards the water and sanitation target', www.tearfund.org.

Toubkiss, J. (2006) 'Costing MDG Target 10 on Water Supply and Sanitation: Comparative Analysis, Obstacles and Recommendations', Marseilles: World Water Council.

Transparency International (2006) *Global Corruption Report 2006 —Special Focus on Corruption and Health*, London: Transparency International.

Transparency International (2005) 'Stealing our future: corruption in the classroom', http://www.transparencia.org.es.

United Nations (a) 'Universal Declaration of Human Rights (UDHR)', www.un.org/Overview/rights.html (last checked by the author March 2006).

United Nations (b) 'Convention on the Rights of the Child (CRC)', www.unhchr.ch/html/menu3/b/k2crc.htm (last checked by the author March 2006).

United Nations (2005) 'Progress Towards the Millennium Development Goals, 1990–2005', http://unstats.un.org/unsd/mi/goals_2005/goal_2.pdf (last checked by the author March 2006).

UNAIDS/ World Health Organisation (2005) 'AIDS Epidemic Update', www.unaids.org/epi/2005/doc/EPIupdate2005_pdf_en/epi-update2005_en.pdf (last checked by the author March 2006).

UNAIDS (2005) 'The "Three Ones" in Action: Where We Are and Where We Go From Here', Geneva: Joint United Nations Programme on HIV/AIDS.

UNAIDS (2004) *2004 Report on the Global AIDS Epidemic*, Geneva: UNAIDS.

UNDP (2005a) *Human Development Report 2005: International Cooperation at a Crossroads: Aid, Trade and Security in an Unequal World*', New York: UNDP.

UNDP (2005b) *Investing in Development: A Practical Plan to Achieve the Millennium Development Goals*, New York, NY: UN Millennium Development Commission.

UNDP (2005c) 'Toward Universal Primary Education; Investments, Incentives, and Institutions', *UN Millennium Project, Taskforce on Education and Gender Equality*, London: UNDP.

UN Department of Economic and Social Affairs (2005a) 'Report on the World Situation', www.un.org/esa/socdev/rwss/docs/Chapter3.pdf (last checked by the author March 2006).

UN Department of Economic and Social Affairs (2005b) 'Progress Towards the Millennium Development Goals, 1990–2005', http://unstats.un.org/unsd/mi/goals_2005/goal_6.doc (last checked by the author March 2006).

UN Department of Economic and Social Affairs 'The Convention on the Elimination of All Forms of Discrimination against Women (CEDAW)', www.un.org/womenwatch/daw/cedaw (last checked by the author March 2006).

UN Economic and Social Council 'General Comment No.15: The right to water (Articles 11 and 12 of the International Covenant on Economic, Social and Cultural Rights)', www.unhchr.ch/html/menu2/6/gc15.doc (last checked by the author March 2006).

UNESCO (2006) *'Education For All Global Monitoring Report 2006: Literacy for Life'*, Paris: UNESCO.

UNESCO (2005a) *'Children out of School: Measuring Exclusion from Primary Education'*, Montreal: UNESCO Institute for Statistics.

UNESCO (2005b) *Global Monitoring Report: Addressing Progress towards the EFA Goals*, New York: UNESCO.

UNESCO (a) 'Education for All: Dakar Framework for Action', www.unesco.org/education/efa/ed_for_all/framework.shtml (last checked by the author March 2006).

UNESCO (b) 'World Declaration for Education for All', www.unesco.org/education/efa/ed_for_all/background/jomtien_declaration.shtml (last checked by the author March 2006).

UNICEF (a) 'Delivery Care', www.childinfo.org/areas/deliverycare/ (last checked by the author March 2006).

UNICEF (b) 'At a Glance: Brazil', www.unicef.org/infobycountry/brazil_statistics.html (last checked by the author March 2006).

USAID (2003) 'The Health Sector Human Resource Crisis in Africa: An Issues Paper', Washington, DC: USAID.

Unsworth, S. (2001) 'Understanding Pro-Poor Change: A Discussion Paper'. Mimeo.

Vidal, J. (2005) 'Flagship water privatisation fails in Tanzania', *Guardian*, 25 May 2005. www.guardian.co.uk/hearafrica05/story/0,15756,1491600,00.html (last checked by the author April 2006).

Vyas, S. and N. Palmer (2005) 'The Non-State Sector and Health — Literature Review and Four-Country Study', background research paper for Oxfam, December 2005.

Wakefield, E. (2004) 'Mapping of Donors' Policies and Approaches to Non-State Service Providers', research commissioned for DFID by International Development Department, University of Birmingham, UK.

WaterAid (2006a) 'Getting the Off-Track "On Target"', a background paper on water and sanitation for the Human Development Report 2006.

WaterAid (2006b) 'Bridging the Gap: Citizens' Action for Accountability in Water and Sanitation', (forthcoming).

WaterAid (2005a) 'Dying for the Toilet', www.un-ngls.org/un-summit-wateraid.pdf (last checked by the author March 2006).

WaterAid (2005b) 'Getting to Boiling Point: Turning up the Heat on Water and Sanitation', London: WaterAid. www.wateraid.org.

WaterAid Nepal (2004) 'The Water and Sanitation Millennium Development Targets in Nepal: What do they mean? What will they cost? Can Nepal meet them?', www.wateraid.org.

WaterAid Nepal (2002) 'Sustained Drinking Water and Sanitation for All in Nepal — Sector Financing Requirement', www.wateraid.org/documents/nepal_sector_financing_requirements.pdf.

Watkins, K. (2006) 'We cannot tolerate children dying for a glass of water', *Guardian,* 8 March 2006, www.guardian.co.uk/water/story/0,,1725920,00.html (last checked by the author March 2006).

Watt, P. (2003) 'Comment on Draft 2004 World Development Report', ActionAid, May 2003 (unpublished).

Watt, P. (2000) *Social Investment and Economic Growth — A Strategy to Eradicate Poverty*, Oxford: Oxfam GB.

Wood, A. (2005a) 'World Bank's Poverty Reduction Support Credit — Continuity or Change?', Dublin: Debt and Development Coalition Ireland, www.debtireland.org/resources/index.htm.

Wood, A. (2005b), 'The Pros and Cons of Old and New Conditionality for Debt Cancellation', Jubilee Debt Campaign, March 2006.

World Bank (2006) *Global Monitoring Report 2006 — Millennium Development Goals: Strengthening Mutual Accountability, Aid, Trade and Governance*, Washington: World Bank.

World Bank (2005a) *Improving Women's Lives: World Bank Actions Since Beijing*, Washington, DC: World Bank Gender and Development Group.

World Bank (2005b) *Global Monitoring Report 2005*, Washington: International Bank for Reconstruction/World Bank.

World Bank (2005c) 'World AIDS Day', www.worldbank.org/worldaidsday/charts.htm (last checked by the author March 2006).

World Bank (2004a) *World Development Report 2004: Making Services Work for Poor People*, Washington, DC: World Bank.

World Bank (2004b) 'EFA Fast-Track Initiative Framework,' www.worldbank.org/education/efafti/documents/Moscow/FTI_Framework_amended_with_gender_specific_out comes_draft_P1.pdf (last checked by the author March 2006).

World Bank Operations Evaluation Department (2002) 'Assessing the World Bank Water Resources Strategy', Washington DC: World Bank.

World Bank (a) 'Education for All Fast-Track Initiative', www.worldbank.org/education/efafti/ (last checked by the author March 2006).

World Bank (2003) 'Issue Brief: User Fees', Washington DC: World Bank.

World Health Organization (2006) *World Health Report 2006 — Working Together for Health*, Geneva: World Health Organization.

World Health Organization (2001) 'Macroeconomics and Health: Investing in Health for Economic Development. Report of the Commission on Macroeconomics and Health', Geneva: WHO.

World Health Organization (a) 'Health Through Safe Drinking Water and Basic Sanitation', www.who.int/water_sanitation_health/mdg1/en/index.html (last checked by the author March 2006).

World Health Organization (b) 'Millennium Development Goals: Goal 4: Reduce Child Mortality', www.who.int/mdg/goals/goal4/en/index.html (last checked by the author March 2006).

Yates, J., R. Cooper and J. Holland (2006) 'Social protection and health: experiences in Uganda', *Development Policy Review*, 2006, 24(3): 339–56.

Yates, R. (2004) 'Should African Governments Scrap User Fees for Health Services?', presentation to Oxfam GB, September 2004.

www.ingramcontent.com/pod-product-compliance
Lightning Source LLC
Jackson TN
JSHW052134131224
75386JS00037B/1265

* 9 7 8 0 8 5 5 9 8 5 6 9 1 *